How Yoga Works

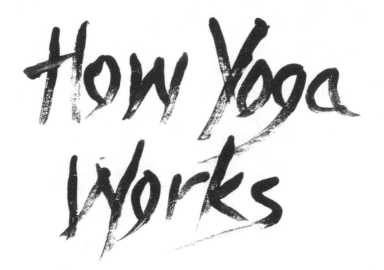

MARK -

LET THESE SEEDS BE A GIFT TO YOU.

CAROLE & JIMMY

Other works by Geshe Michael Roach:

The Diamond Cutter: The Buddha on Managing Your Business and Your Life

The Garden: A Parable

The Tibetan Book of Yoga: Ancient Buddhist Teachings on the Philosophy and Practice of Yoga

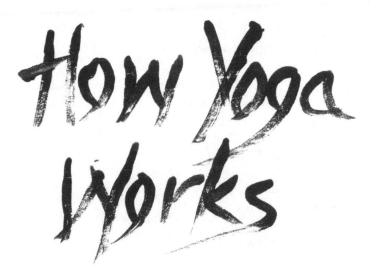

How Yoga Works

Healing Yourself and Others with the Yoga Sutra

Geshe Michael Roach

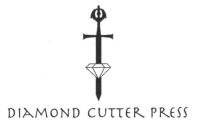

DIAMOND CUTTER PRESS

Published in 2004 by Diamond Cutter Press

Cover design by Geshe Michael Roach
Interior design by Clare Cerullo

Printed in the United States of America

Library of Congress Cataloging-in-Publication Data

Roach, Michael, 1952-
 How yoga works : healing yourself and others with the Yoga sutra
/ by Geshe Michael Roach and Christie McNally with the Diamond
Mountain Teachers, Debra Ballier ... [et al.].
    p. cm.
 In English; includes translations from Sanskrit.
 ISBN 1-57467-105-7
 1. Yoga. I. McNally, Christie. II. Ballier, Debra. III. Patañjali. Yogasutra.
English. Selections. IV. Diamond Mountain Teachers. V. Title.

B132.Y6R6 2004
181'.452--dc22
                    2004014727

www.diamondcutterpress.com

Table of Contents

1   THE PLACE WE ALL START FROM   1

2   WELL-BEING THAT STAYS   11

3   A REASON NOT TO SKIP   17

4   A BALANCE OF FEELINGS   23

5   DOING IT RIGHT   28

6   THE HARASSMENT OF PREFERENCES   32

7   CULTIVATING THE PRACTICE   37

8   CHANNELS OF LIGHT   44

9   NORTH STAR   54

10   HORSES AND HORSEMEN   59

11   BREATH AND A SMILE   67

12   BREATH AND HEART   75

13   SILENT SITTING   80

14   LEARNING HOW TO SIT   86

15   FREE KINDNESS   92

16   WE MISUNDERSTAND OUR WORLD   99

17   THE PEN AGAIN   106

18   OUT THERE, OVER THERE   114

19   EVEN FOR THOSE WHO UNDERSTAND   119

20   FIST AND LIGHTNING   124

21   TRULY, EVERYTHING IS SUFFERING   129

22   A VESSEL   132

23   PRIDE BEFORE A FALL   140

24   NEXT TO GODLINESS   148

25   TWO INVITATIONS   158

26   FLESH OR LIGHT   171

27   SEEDS, AND NOT DECISIONS   181

28   SEEDS ARE PLANTED   186

29	THE FIRST QUESTION	197
30	THE GARDENING BEGINS	206
31	BREAKING THE CIRCLE	215
32	THE FORTRESS OF LITTLE THINGS	224
33	DIFFICULT QUESTIONS AND DIFFICULT ANSWERS	235
34	WORLDVIEW	249
35	MATCHING PICTURES	262
36	PLANTING HIGHER SEEDS	271
37	JOY	283
38	TAKING NOT THINKING	288
39	BEGINNING THE END OF OLD BAD SEEDS	298
40	OLD DEBTS CANCELLED	313
41	THE SPIRIT'S BREATH	322
42	SEEDS OF THOUGHT	332
43	EASY POINTS	337
44	THE SEER DWELLS	343
45	TIME AND SPACE, REDUCED TO A PUDDLE	352
46	STANDING ON THE RIVER	373
47	GRACE	389
48	YOUR HAND	403

1

The Place We All Start From

Third Week of February,
Iron Snake Year (1101 A.D.)

It was just another one of those dusty little Indian towns. No sign before, no way to even know what they call it—the road just starts to get wider, and you see more people on it, and then suddenly the wild green of the jungle ends, and you spot the first little houses of brown mud brick. And then you're in a little stream of farmers, and women carrying water in clay jugs on their heads, and cows and pigs and chickens, all headed for the middle of town.

We came to a stout wood pole stretched across the road, about waist high. There was a little guardhouse set up on the side, with a bored policeman leaning out a small window in the heat of the sun and the dust of the road. Long-Life and I had seen dozens of little checkpoints like this in the past year—the police were supposed to catch people poaching wood or wild animals from the jungle, which was the property of whatever little local tyrant called himself King. Mostly though the police simply took the opportunity to force bribes out of travelling merchants.

People and animals just came up to the pole and ducked under and went on, and so Long-Life and I did too. It was easier for Long-Life, you see. He's a little Tibetan moustache dog, about as high as your ankles.

As we went under, the policeman stepped out. He leaned over lazily and picked up a stone and threw it at Long-Life, who was used to this greeting in India and dodged it easily. But I was tired and hot, and threw an insolent glance at the man as I collected Long-Life in my arms.

"You," he called.

I walked on without a pause, something my grandmother had taught me. You could always say you hadn't heard.

"You there. Stop." And then the sound of a *lathi* tapped on the ground. A *lathi* is a strong, flexible, wicked wooden stick; if you put one end on the ground the other comes up to about your waist, and all the policemen carry one. It doesn't look like much, but in the right hands it can lay your skin open in a minute. And some of these men, I knew, were really looking for an excuse to use it. And so I stopped.

"Come back here." I turned, and looked at his face. Dark with hours in the sun, and dark with an evil temper, and something else. I walked back slowly, trying to look calm.

"Into the guardhouse," he ordered, pointing with his stick. It was hardly big enough for a single person, let alone the two of us. But better not to fight; the fingers around the stick were tensed.

He pushed in after me, too close, and then I knew what it was about him. He had that sweet stench of a man who drank too much of the local sugarcane liquor. He leered at me with his bloodshot eyes, up and down the simple pink-hued orange of the light cotton *sari* dress I'd traded for my warm mountain woolens, nearly a year ago.

"You're not from around here," he said, almost accusing me.

"No sir, I am not."

"Then where are you from?"

"From Tibet," I said. He looked at me blankly. "The snow mountains," I added, pointing vaguely off to the north.

He nodded, but his eyes were already down, crudely across my chest, then to Long-Life, and then to my red woolen bag.

"What's in the bag?" he said, again in that policeman's accusation. I'd heard it too a hundred times. The preliminary to a demand for a bribe.

I was in no mood. "Nothing of value," I replied, trying to inch a little further back from his body, and his stink.

"Open it," he ordered, pointing to a little shelf at the window, near our elbows.

I gave him one hard glance and silently set my things out on the shelf. All my things in the world: a shawl from Katrin; a small wooden bowl; and the book, wrapped against the weather.

"Open it," he demanded, pointing to the book. I opened the wrapping, and he leaned over the ancient pages, as if to read them. They were upside down.

"It is old," he declared, standing straight again, glaring into my eyes.

"It is," I said simply.

"Where did you get it?"

"My Teacher gave it to me," I replied.

He looked in my face again. "Your teacher," he said in disbelief.

"My Teacher," I repeated.

"Put it back," he said, waving to the book and my things. I collected them slowly, trying not to let him see that my hands were shaking. I looked past him, out the door.

"Then may I go, sir?"

3

He took the bag from my hands. "You will come with me," and he turned and walked down the road, to the town.

I followed behind, my heart pounding and Long-Life pressed to my chest. In about half an hour the man turned off the road into a dusty little yard. At the back there was a dirty, shabby building of the same dull brown mud brick. It had a porch with a thatched palm cover, fallen down on one side, thick with the hot dry dirt of the yard. At the very top of the building, scratched across the mud, was the face of a lion with two swords crossed below it. Sign of the local king, I thought to myself—they're all pretty much the same. At least he hadn't taken me home. Maybe I could talk to someone higher up, someone who wasn't drunk.

The dark man stepped to the side and pointed to the door with his stick. "Inside," he grunted.

I held up my skirt and stepped across the dirt piled up on the porch, then through a small door.

"Sit down," he said, pointing to a little wooden bench against the wall. He turned into a doorway opposite the bench, and I could hear him talking to someone there in low tones.

I surveyed the little police station, the jail, for now I could see what it was. I sat in a largish room; the back was divided into three crude cells of the same mud brick. The front of each cell was open to view, with stout bamboo bars from ceiling to floor, and a little door of the same material. Two cells were empty, but in the one to the right there was a figure lying face down on the bare floor.

The wall across from me had a rack of old, rusted swords and spears, locked across with a bar. The real weapons—for major trouble, something this town had probably never seen. And then two small rooms behind where I was sitting, and that was it. My eyes returned to the floor, and the same piles of dirt.

The policeman came back out. "Come," he ordered again, pointing to the door behind him. I entered with an uneasy feeling, clutching Long-Life tightly.

"Sit down," he said again, pointing this time to a grass mat on the floor. "The Captain wants to talk to you. Wait." And he was gone, and the door was closed.

I sat and looked at the Captain. He was seated on a thicker mat and cushions at the head of the room, bent over a low table covered with papers, seeming to be quite occupied writing something out with a bamboo pen. But I knew this little bureaucrat's trick too by now. He would let me wait, until he was sure I was uncomfortable, before he even acknowledged that I was there. It was a way of saying that I was beneath his notice.

And so I took the time to study the room, and the Captain too. He was surrounded in disorder, stacks of ledgers and papers, everything covered with the same brown dust. The only light was from a small window across from the door, but the afternoon sun lay across him and his work.

I guessed he was about 35, the career public servant type, settled into his middle age. I think at one time he must have been handsome: he had thick black hair, coming out in little curls, but peppered now with gray—too early gray, I thought. When he looked to the side and checked some list of things I could see him flinch slightly—with that and his stooped shoulders I guessed he had hurt his back from years of sitting like this in his office, hunched over his reports. His face had been strong, I think, almost noble; but now it was marred by lines of pain cutting down between his eyebrows, and crossing the corners of his mouth. His cheeks had gone a little puffy, and there were bags under his eyes—

probably having trouble sleeping, with the pain in his back, and some other pain too; something in his heart, I thought. And then not to seem too forward I lowered my eyes again, and waited, as a woman in those times was expected to.

Finally he set his pen down and covered his ink pot, and raised his eyes to me, with the steadiness of authority.

"The Sergeant says I should waste my time questioning a girl with a book," he sighed.

I looked up and gazed into his face. It was not an unkind face, but it was the face of someone in pain, and so I thought it better to be quiet. There was a pause, and in that one moment I felt him ready to send me on my way. I looked to the door, and he seemed to hesitate, but then when I looked back he was studying my face, as if I were someone he might have known. Then he looked down for a moment, and set his hand on the little writing desk.

"Come here, closer. Show me the book."

I moved up across from him, took the book from my bag, and set it on the desk. I went to open it but his hands were already there, strong handsome hands, and he unwrapped it with a quick gesture. He knew about books.

"The Sergeant was right," he nodded. "It is old—the old kind, letters scratched into palm leaf."

I nodded, my heart sinking.

"How did you get this book?" he said, looking stern now into my face.

"My Teacher gave it to me."

"Teacher? What kind of teacher?"

"The one, sir," and now I knew it could be trouble, but as always I knew it was better to be honest, "the one who . . . who taught it to me."

"*Taught* it to you?"

"Yes, sir."

"To you, to a girl? How old are you?"

"Seventeen, sir."

"And you . . . you have studied a book like this?"

"I have," I replied, raising my head with some pride, as Grandmother would have.

"Where?"

"In my own country, in Tibet."

"And that is where your teacher is?"

"Yes sir . . . or . . ."

"Or what?"

"Where my Teacher was . . ."

"He is dead?"

"My Teacher is . . ." How could he ever understand? "My Teacher is . . . is gone."

"Gone?" he was staring at me now, alert, sensing the hesitation.

"Yes sir," I said, settling back, starting to worry now.

"And why then have you come to India?"

"I am travelling to the Ganges River, to Varanasi, to study further there."

"Study? A girl? Study with whom?"

"With a Teacher there," I replied, lamely.

"What teacher? What is his name?"

"I don't know . . ."

"Don't know? How will you find him?"

Or her? I thought, but all I could do was shake my head.

He was searching my face again. "How long have you been travelling?"

I looked up at the ceiling and counted the months. "A year, sir. Almost exactly a year."

"And what does your husband think of this?"

"I . . . I have no husband, sir."

"Your father, then."

"My father . . . my father knows I have come to India."

"Knows but not approved?" he retorted, and all I could do was look at the floor.

The Captain sighed again, and ran his finger along the title of the book. I could see his lips moving, working out the sounds of the Sanskrit, the Mother Tongue, written there. And so he can read it, I thought, but only barely — only just the sounds.

"It is the *Yoga Sutra,*" he said softly. "The great Mother of all the teachings on yoga."

I nodded.

"And you know it? Do you know it well?"

I nodded again.

He straightened up suddenly in his seat, and I saw him wince again, so used to it that he was not even aware he was wincing.

"Imagine how it all sounds to me," he said. "A girl, a girl your age, claiming to know a book like this, a priceless book, learned from a missing teacher. And wandering around a foreign country alone, with no husband, without her father's permission, headed for a teacher with no name. And, if the Sergeant is to be believed, without a penny in her possession."

I nodded. This was the sum of my life.

"And so you swear the book is your own? You have not stolen it?"

"It is mine."

He sighed again, heavily, and then suddenly turned the book around towards me. He flipped through several palm-leaf pages and pulled them off, then stabbed his finger at a page.

"Here then, here. Read what is says right here."

I leaned over the desk. "It is from the second chapter," I began. "And it says:

> *Things that cannot last*
> *Seem to us as if they will.*
>
> II.5A"

The Captain's eyes suddenly dropped, and stayed there a moment. When he looked up they were glistening, as though he were about to cry. And there was an anger, or perhaps an anguish, in his voice.

"What does that mean?" he demanded.

"It is talking about our lives," I replied quietly. "Our friends, our family, our work, our own bodies. When they are there, in front of us—when we can see them, and touch them—it seems as though they will always be there. But then they always leave us."

His face tightened. "That is not what is says."

"It is, most certainly, exactly what it says, sir."

"You are lying. You are just making something up, trying to get away with this thing, this thing you have stolen. But that is not what the book says. This is a book about yoga, the greatest book of yoga—and yoga is . . . yoga is, well, you know—exercises, things you do, special exercises, to get healthy, to fix problems, problems like with your body." And he leaned towards me intensely, and it made him wince again, unaware of it still.

"That *is* what it says," I repeated.

The Captain glared at me, and closed the book. I reached out to wrap it, but his hand came down on the pages, hard.

"I will keep this," he said flatly.

"But I need it."

"Maybe so, but no matter. You are staying too."

My mouth fell open, and tears of rage and fear welled up, despite myself.

The Captain stood up, with some difficulty, staring down at me.

"We will see if anyone reports the book stolen. It may take . . . some days. During that time you will have a chance to prove that the book is really yours."

"But . . . but how?" I cried.

"Easy," he smiled, but with a shadow of tension. "I have a problem, you see. I have hurt my back; it has hurt . . . for a long time. And yoga, yoga, I know, would fix it. And so it is easy, you see. You will show me how to fix my back; and if you succeed, then I will know that you know yoga, and I can believe that the book is yours. Understood?" he said, with finality.

"But . . . ," I said.

"Sergeant," he called to the door. "Come and lock her up."

2

Well-Being
That Stays

Fourth Week of February

The Sergeant led me roughly by the arm to the middle cell, pushed me inside, and barred the door. A moment later he was back with a stout piece of rope.

"Tie it around the dog's neck."

"He stays with me," I said, trying to muster Grandmother's tone of authority, but failing.

"No dogs in the jail," he answered simply. I stood without moving, and glared at him, and then simply cried. It worked, a bit.

"Going to tie him up outside," said the Sergeant, trying to sound gruff. "You'll be able to see him, out the window." He pointed his stick to the back wall, to a small window with bars.

"And food? And water?" I asked.

He looked at me with a dark amusement. "Same as you," he said simply. He tapped the stick impatiently on the floor, and I realized I was lucky he wasn't just going to kill Long-Life. I stooped and tied the rope, and told my little lion to go along with it all—this was not the time for removing chunks of flesh from people's legs. He was calm and seemed to understand; we had been through a lot together, and this was just one more thing to bear for our larger goal. And so he went.

I could see him then out the window, and as dusk settled we discovered a little hole down at the bottom of the wall. I could reach out and touch Long-Life's nose if we both stretched, but the brick there was all covered with filth. I stood up tall at the window and peeked down, and saw a little trench dug down the back of the cell, ending in a stagnant pool of stench at the edge of the building. Then I realized that this little hole was to be my toilet, and I turned and looked back out the front of the cell.

The Sergeant was still there, sitting on the bench, his eyes glued on me mercilessly, with a kind of hunger—the kind he might show for a jar of liquor. And suddenly I saw that this would be the most terrible part of the jail—to be on display, to be stared at, all day, and all night, by anyone who wished to stare, whether I was awake, or sleeping, or even going to the bathroom.

At first I determined that they should never see anything, but then I sat and thought about what my Teacher would have done: what Katrin would have done. The words of the Master, the words of Patanjali, who a thousand years before had written the little book on the Captain's desk, came to mind, in my Teacher's voice:

> *And they realize that*
> *The body itself is a prison.*
>
> III.39B

In a way, I thought, we are all in a prison, a prison from which only death can release us. And these other prisons—

well—then they are just a point of view. I had a wonderful chance here to make myself stronger, and perhaps to help others—the other people here, including the Sergeant, each in a jail of their own. And so I simply laid down on some straw piled in a corner, and took my rest.

φ

I woke at the usual time, before dawn, and went through all my regular morning practices. I had learned a long time before that keeping them up every day was more important than the problems that would always arise and try to stop them. Thankfully the jail was dark, and the only sound was the gentle snoring of the man on the floor in the next cell. At least he wasn't dead.

Afterwards I sat and thought for a while. I thought about the Captain, and his bad back. I could think of all this as something terrible, as something that could even cost Long-Life and myself our lives, or I could try to see if perhaps something bigger was happening.

I began to think of the best and fastest way I could help the Captain cure his bad back, and it occurred to me that events had thrust me to the very place I had always said I wanted to go: to an opportunity where I could help others heal themselves, with the knowledge of yoga—the knowledge of the Master's little book. And then I caught myself thinking like my Teacher, appreciating for the very first time what it must have been like to stand on the other side, looking at a student like myself. It dawned on me suddenly that the job of teaching me, so full of pride and stubbornness, had surely been more difficult than fixing a tired office worker's bad back. And so I began to make my plans.

The sun was well up by the time anything stirred in the jail. First a tall, younger man came through the front door, and then simply turned around, leaned against the door frame, and stood there, staring out at the people passing on the road. About ten minutes later the Captain came up the path and onto the porch; the younger man straightened up sharply, saluted, and stepped to the side respectfully as his superior entered.

The Captain waved at my cell. "Bring the prisoner to my room." The younger man turned and, with a look of surprise, saw me for the first time. He came and collected me quietly, took me to the Captain, and then left and closed the door.

"We will begin now," the Captain commanded.

I nodded. "Please come and stand here," I said, pointing to the middle of the room. He came, and stood, and I looked him over silently, as my Teacher had me that first day. And then I knew what Katrin had been looking at, because the very way the Captain stood there told me everything about his life.

His tummy and chin and skin were loose, with that look of a person who works at a desk all day. His shoulders were bent in, and his neck looked frozen in place, from years of tension—trying to please his own superiors, wherever they were. And the pain in the back and the pain of his life were making his once-gentle features hard and lined.

I could see the layers of him: body sagging and locking up; the joints inside stiffening; the inner winds choked at the joints; his thoughts strangling the inner winds; the troubles of his life disturbing his thoughts; and the very source of all the events of his life at the very middle of it all—each one caused by the other, and nothing he could stop by himself, because he didn't even know it was happening.

But where to start with him? Where would my Teacher have started with him? I heard Katrin's voice again, and I spoke the words of the Master out loud to the Captain, to my very first pupil:

> *"The poses bring a feeling of well-being*
> *Which stays with you.*
>
> II.46"

"The poses—you mean, the exercises?" he said. "Now that sounds more like yoga."

I smiled. "It is where we will begin, at least. Now stand as straight as you can . . . ," and I spent an hour just getting him to stand in his body the way he was meant to stand in his body; the way he had stood in it before, before his habits had bent and twisted his frame. And then so he wouldn't think I didn't know anything more, I took him through what we call Bowing to the Sun, which left him puffing within a few minutes.

At the end he had a look of accomplishment—the same look I must have had on the first day, I realized, and I knew he deserved it. It takes so much courage just to start, I thought.

"Now I want you to do this much every morning for the next week," I said. "It's just five or ten minutes. And then we will go on from there. The poses will fix your back—just like the book says," I nodded pointedly to my book, still in the center of his desk. "It will cure your back, and cure it for good."

The Captain nodded happily, and sent me back to my cell.

φ

Around noon on that first day, a small boy appeared in the doorway of the jail. He was thin and barefoot, dressed only in a ragged pair of shorts. In his hands he held a tray covered with a cloth; he went to one of the rooms on the side, and then came back out with the younger policeman. They went to the cell next to mine, and I could hear the door there open, and then the boy left. The smell of fresh rice and handmade bread wafted towards me, and I realized Long-Life and I hadn't eaten for a day or two.

We were used to this on the road, eating only when we found some fruit in the trees, or a stranger who was willing to share some scraps of a meal. But the smell was overwhelming. I waited for my own meal to come, and then suddenly realized there might be no meal. And just as suddenly a hand reached around from the other cell, and pushed a small cup of rice and beans in, between the bars.

"Eat," a voice whispered from the other side of the wall. "Fast, then push the cup back. And for heaven's sake don't let the Sergeant see you." I gulped the food down, setting aside a good part to hand through to Long-Life, and got the cup back just before the Sergeant's shadow loomed in the front door.

3

A Reason
Not to Skip

First Week of March

It always surprises me how fast we get used to something. The days passed, and I made good use of them, settling down into a routine of yoga and a silent mental review of the lessons that Katrin had taught me. And so it was as if I'd gone on a retreat, which I suppose I had. Life in the dirty little jail outside was dull—only an occasional farmer coming in to report a stolen cow, things like that. The cups from the other side of the wall came silently, every day, always right after one of the young boys delivered a fresh tray next door. It was just barely enough for Long-Life and I, and the younger policeman left me a small jug of water each morning. I handed palmfuls out through the filthy hole to Long-Life, who was panting from the heat, tied to a barren tree. Long before I had cut his luxurious hair short, so he could travel better in the Indian sun—but he was suffering.

The next class with the Captain was exactly a week from the first. He had me brought into his office, and I asked him to repeat what he had learned. After a minute or two I could see he had missed three, maybe even four days of practice. I stopped him.

"You've been skipping your practice," I said firmly. "And the Master says, in my book over there on your desk, that:

> *Your practice must be steady,*
> *Without gaps.*
>
> I.14B"

"I didn't skip my practice," he replied, in a voice that said he was unaccustomed to being challenged. But I knew I had to press the point, now, or he would never be healed.

"You did," I repeated. "I can see it, as plain as day, the way you can probably look into . . . into a real criminal's eyes, and see if he's done something wrong or not."

"I mean to say," the Captain cleared his throat, "that I didn't *skip* a day—I found it *necessary* to *not* do my practice, on a day."

"On *a* day?" I smiled wryly, with a little pang in my heart; for I suddenly recalled Katrin saying the same words to me, with the same smile.

"Perhaps . . . perhaps it was more than that," he allowed.

"Then you must give me back my book now, and let me leave," I said evenly. "Your back will never be healed, if you won't practice steadily, a little every day. The Master himself says,

> *And the fifth of the obstacles*
> *Is laziness.*
>
> I.30E"

The Captain's face clouded; he snapped up straight, with his usual grimace.

"It was *not* laziness!" he retorted. "I am not a lazy person! It was . . . work! Pressing work! I have responsibilities, you know!"

"Always that?" I answered coolly. "Always that? Something important you had to do?"

He paused and seemed to think it over. "And one day—I think it was one day—I really wasn't in the mood, you see? Stretching and bending and groaning and all that; a man my age, with my responsibilities . . ."

"Enough," I smiled, holding up my hand. "I've heard all this before."

"You have?" he looked at me intently. "You have taught many others? I thought . . . I thought that I might be the first."

"Oh, not that I've heard these excuses from others," I laughed. "It's just that I tried to use all of them with my own Teacher, and I know what they are. They are just plain laziness; laziness, don't call it anything more noble. Something else comes up, and the yoga takes a little effort, and time, and so you skip it. You don't really want to do it. You don't really want to heal your back. You should just let me go."

"But I do want it . . . I do want it to be healed. It hurts, you know." He put his hand to his back, and looked down at the floor with a sadness. "It all . . . hurts. I really thought you might be able to help."

We stood there quiet for a while; I looked at him standing like that, in his sadness. It came to me that perhaps he was ready for a bigger step, a step that would take him a long way, if he would really try it.

"Captain, sir, I believe you. I believe that you really want to be healed."

He looked up and gazed at me gently, with a kind of gratitude.

"And so I will tell you something now, something special; it is a little early to tell you, but if you follow it— follow it sincerely—you will be able to practice steadily. You will not skip your practice. And then it will work."

He nodded. "Then tell me. I will try."

I nodded back. "In the book, the Master says again,

And if you wish to stop these obstacles,
There is one, and only one,
Crucial practice for doing so.
                    I.32"

"And what is that?" he asked.

"And then the Master says,

You must use compassion.
                    I.33B"

The Captain turned and gazed out the window. "Compassion? What's that supposed to mean? How would that stop me from skipping my practice?"

"It's something you have to understand," I said quietly. "It's something important. You see, you can't do this, you can't do yoga, just to fix your own back. It's too small. We are too small. If we do something just to help ourselves, it will never work. You can never really put effort into a thing if it's only for yourself. It has to be for something bigger."

"Bigger? Like what?"

"Look at the way a woman will work for her children— look at the work they can do, twenty-four hours a day, day in and day out, for ten, twenty years. It puts your little office work to shame. And they can do it for only one reason—

because they are not doing it only for themselves. They are doing it for others too."

The Captain laughed. "So you want me to do my yoga for other people too? Are you telling me I won't be able to fix my back unless I figure out how to fix a couple of other backs along the way?"

"Something like that," I said. "All you really have to do is think about helping some other people with what you learn. If I taught you all this yoga and suddenly your back got better and you were walking around with a big smile on your face all the time, would it do anything, say, for the Sergeant, or for that younger policeman?"

"For the corporal?" the Captain smiled. "I don't know—it would take a lot to get him to do anything. He never has any energy; he never gets excited about anything. He eats a pile of his mother's buttered flatbreads—fills up that little pot belly—and strolls to work. Then he stands at the door there and stares out at nothing all day." He paused. "But could yoga do anything for him? Do you think it could give him a little pep, a little interest in his life?"

"It does a lot of things," I replied, "a lot of things you can hardly guess. But yes, certainly, it would change his life." I paused myself, so he'd listen to what came next. "But you see, in a way, now that he knows you've started yoga, he'll wait and see if it helps you. If it obviously does, then we could get him to fix himself. And so you see, if you have compassion—if you keep thinking that if you fix your back you might also be fixing the corporal—then when a day comes that you feel like skipping your practice, you won't. Because you'd be hurting him, you see?"

The Captain mulled this over, but I could see the idea might not be clear enough in his heart to work. And just

21

then the door to his office burst open, and there was the Sergeant, panting for breath, his face red and contorted from his liquor.

"Oh!" he exclaimed. "Sorry sir! Didn't know you were . . . er . . . occupied!" He stood there stupidly, weaving in the doorway, leering at the two of us.

"That too?" said the Captain to me, quietly.

"Same thing," I replied.

He nodded. "I won't forget." And then, "Sergeant, could you help the prisoner back to her cell?"

4

A Balance
of Feelings

Second Week of March

More days flew by. Long-Life's rope stretched out and he
could get up closer to the little hole, and I could scratch his
head a bit. I began to work out the schedule kept by my
three captors: the Captain followed typical office hours,
wandering in by mid-morning, doing some work, taking a
long lunch, then talking with a few friends who came, taking
tea, a touch of work, and then off to home. The Sergeant and
the corporal divided up the day, and one always slept in the
side room at night.

One night there was a little commotion—someone
banged on the front door and woke up the Sergeant, and he
had to leave with them, barring the door on the way out. A
few minutes later there was a tap from the cell next door.

"Girl," the man said. "Girl, are you awake?"

I was a little stunned. I had given up hope of having
anyone to talk to. "Yes, yes I am."

"Good, good. We should talk a bit. But careful you listen
well for the door. The prisoners are absolutely forbidden to

talk, and the Sergeant will flay the skin off our backs with that idiot stick of his if he catches us. Got it?"

"Oh yes," I said, then suddenly at a loss for words.

"What's your name?" he whispered.

It dawned on me that no one here had even asked me that yet. "Why, it's Friday," I whispered back. "My name is Friday."

"Born on a Friday, yes?" he whispered.

"Yes, yes that . . . and more."

"Well I'm Busuku," he whispered back, stretching out the sounds, *boo-soo-koo*.

"Busuku?" I said. "Sounds like a nice name. Does it have a meaning?"

"Oh yes," he replied with a chuckle. "It means 'Mister Worthless.' I guess a lot of people figure I'm the most worthless person in this worthless little town."

"Well, I don't think so. I don't know what we would have done without you."

"We? Oh—you're giving some of the food to the dog."

"Oh yes, but—not just a dog, you see . . . "

"I understand. So I'll send a bit more. But we have to talk . . . ," and then the front door burst open, and I could see the Sergeant's form there, and we froze. But he just mumbled something to himself and stumbled to his room, and all was quiet again.

ϕ

The next time the Captain called me in he remained at his little desk, and waved me to the mat on the floor in front of him.

"Something's wrong," he said.

"What's that?"

"I did what you said — what the book said, or what you say the book says. Anyway I've been able to practice every single day, except my day off . . . " He looked up at me like a schoolboy, to see if he was in trouble.

"A day off is fine," I said. "That's not skipping, if you choose a regular day or two of the week to rest from your practice. That's perfect."

"Yes, well—I'm glad, I thought so. And you're right, just thinking of the corporal, and the Sergeant . . . " He stopped suddenly, and turned and gazed out the window for a moment. Then he turned back and looked at me.

"They are in such pain, you know—just normal people, trying to live their lives—but everybody has something. It took me a long time to realize that. And so thinking I might help them, even a little, it has worked, you know. I haven't skipped a day. But now I don't think it's going to work out."

"Why not?"

"Well you see, once I started to do the yoga every day, even just a little a day, well then you see I started to hurt all over. And my bones, you see—my knees, and my arms, and sometimes my back—they make these popping sounds when I do the exercises. And so, you see, maybe I'm different—maybe this isn't going to work for me." He looked at me a little crestfallen.

"Popping sounds?" I said. "Little cracking sounds, as if you were cracking your fingers?"

"Just so!" he exclaimed.

I smiled. "That's very normal, especially for a man your age. The joints between the bones, you see—especially in your knees, or your neck, your back and shoulder—they have been freezing up, more and more each year. You probably hardly noticed it. And now we are opening them back up, releasing little places where the inner winds have locked up, and it makes that little sound. But you should let me know right away if anything else happens that actually hurts."

He nodded, but his mind had gone on. "Inner winds?" he asked.

"Later," I replied. "Later. Right now you should be happy when you hear that noise. And as the joints open up and the winds begin to flow again, it will go away. You won't even notice when it does."

"But what about the rest?" he insisted. "You're supposed to be fixing me! But I get up out of bed and walk to the station like a duck, I'm so sore!"

I laughed again. Just to imagine I had bothered my Teacher too with all this silly talk, almost the very same words even. "You are sore," I said, "because you are waking up muscles that have slept a long time; and if you don't wake them up your back will never get better. That's what holds your back up in the first place. And when you feel a little sore like this I want you to remember something else from the Master's *Short Book about Yoga*. It says,

> *Learn to keep your feelings in balance,*
> *Whether something feels good,*
> *Or whether it hurts.*
>
> I.33D

The point is, there are going to be days when you feel a little sore, and other days when you suddenly make a breakthrough, and it feels great. That's just the way it is, it's the way everything is. And you have to try not to get too discouraged, and not to get too excited, because for the time being things like this will continue to go up and down. You can't let it distract you. You have a goal—you have your two men to think of."

The Captain straightened up, and stood up. He did look sore as he did so, but he didn't wince—although he didn't notice that. He came and I took him through his paces, adding some standing poses like the Triangle to begin building up some strength throughout his body. In one way or another it would all help his back.

When we finished he was sweating but looked invigorated—in his heart as well as his face. He stood there for a minute before sending me back to the cell.

"Something you said," he remarked.

"Yes?"

"You said things would go . . . that they would continue to go up and down. But then you said, 'for the time being.' What's that supposed to mean?"

"It's coming," I smiled. Something Katrin always used to say to me.

5

Doing it Right

Third Week of March

People think jails are bad because you can't go outside when you want to. But I guess if you could ask all the prisoners there ever were the worst thing about being behind bars, it would have to be the ticks—with the fleas running a close second, and then the more occasional visitors like rats and huge jungle cockroaches. The floor was too cold not to sleep on the hay, but the hay was where the ticks slept too.

It wasn't too bad while I was asleep, just a little itching here and there that sent my dreams off on odd detours. But then when the sunlight started to filter in through my window I'd see two or three of the ticks hanging on the wall—where they seemed to prefer to do their digesting— bloated into red sacks the size of a thumbnail, gorged with my blood. And then I'd get rashes that the fleas would find, and both Long-Life and I spent a good deal of our time just sitting and scratching.

The Captain called me in a few days early, which I'd expected. He was starting to feel better, although he still hadn't noticed it himself, and now that he was regular at his practice he had begun to take a little well-deserved pride in it. I watched with satisfaction as he went through his routine—still only about ten minutes of it—but then he reached something called the Western Stretch, where you sit on the floor with your legs stretched out and try to hold your toes.

"Captain. Wait. Stop."

He glanced up at me, his cheek grazing his knee.

"Stop? This is one of my best poses!"

"Yes, best, because you're doing it wrong."

"Certainly not!" he exclaimed, sitting up again. "Why I can already touch my head to my knees!"

"Touch it to your knees, yes, but only because you are cheating; your knees are bent nearly in half! I told you they had to be straight! Now the Master says . . . "

"Master says! Master says! Doesn't the Master ever say I did something right?" he whined.

"The Master says," I repeated with a grin, recalling my tussles with Katrin, "that

> *Your practice must be done correctly,*
> *For then a firm foundation is laid.*
>
> I.14c

You see, the point is not what the pose looks like in the end, to someone watching you—the Captain touching his head to his knees. It's the process of the pose as it goes on, it's what it does inside of you: how it works to begin to straighten and open your channels."

"Channels?" he asked.

"Later!" I said, feeling more and more like grumpy old Katrin. "But if you don't do the pose right, if you cheat, if you try to trick the pose and get around it just so you look good, then the pose doesn't work on you the way it's supposed to. Now try it again. Without bending your knees."

The Captain moaned but stuck out his legs once more. He reached his hands forward towards the vicinity of his shins, then curled his back up like a turtle and plopped his head on his knees.

"No!" I cried, giving his back a little slap—something Katrin would have done to me a dozen times a day.

He was up on his feet in a flash, red in the face, glaring at me. "Why! But! You! What are you doing, you . . . you . . . *girl!*"

"I may be a girl, but I'm still your teacher. You did it wrong again, you did the same thing again. You cheated it. But this time you might have hurt yourself. I told you, the back has to be straight; it *must* be straight. And you bend at the hips, you fold there at the hips, like a hinge—never curl your lower back like that. You'll hurt it, hurt it more. You have to learn to listen to me, you have to do it right, just like the Master says."

He stayed there for a moment, his eyes on me with anger, and then finally let his breath out in a huge sigh.

"All right, look. Suppose I do it your way," he said, sitting down again. "I stick my legs out, very straight. No cheating, you see!" he exclaimed, holding up his arms.

"So far, so good."

"And now I keep my back *very straight*!" he bellowed. "And I *fold*, at my *hips*, like a *hinge*, and then . . ." He bent forward. It looked great.

"You see?" he cried. "You see?"

"See what?" I said.

He pointed to his forehead, and then touched his knees, and held his hands out, frustrated. "My head! It's a good two feet from my knees!"

"And that's fine," I said. "It's what you can do now, if you do it right. And that lays a firm foundation to build from, healing your back all the way. We are here to make you healthy again, not to make sure you can touch your head to your knees."

The Captain shrugged, still a little put out, but then he did the pose right. He really was an intelligent and sensitive man, no matter how hard he tried to hide it.

I gave him some more seated poses, to bring his back along slowly, and then some very gentle twists at the waist, warning him to do only a few, exactly as I'd shown him to. At the end I had him lie quietly and rest for a while, in a pose of perfect quiet and stillness—so still that we call it the Dead Man's Pose. And when he sat up again, he had a question ready for me.

"But you know," he said, "I've watched you do some of the poses. And I know that even if I try I can't really do them right, not the way you do them."

"Oh yes, I know. It's one of the paradoxes of yoga. To really do a pose right you have to do it a little wrong, a thousand times."

"So you can say that doing a pose wrong helps you do a pose right," he concluded cheerfully.

"Not if what you're doing wrong is something your teacher has already corrected," I shot back at him, the way Katrin would have. And he sent me to my cell.

6

The Harassment
of Preferences

Fourth Week of March

After over a month in the dirty little jail I'd worked out small routines to deal with things that you just take for granted elsewhere. Like washing.

My dress was sticky with dust and sweat, and I had developed an odor that I could smell even over the stink of the trench outside my window. The Sergeant didn't seem to have any intention of allowing me enough water to wash myself, and I still found him staring at me in a way that was frightening, especially when he was really drunk. It was as though he was pushing things, waiting for something to happen.

But I figured out a way to take a tiny bit of water each day, and set it in a little depression in the back corner of the cell, where it was cooler, and cover it with hay. After a few days of this I had a large cupful there, and then at night when everything was dark and quiet I'd wash a part of me, or a little section of my dress.

Underneath I always wore a special white cotton loincloth that the sages of the way of yoga wear, something

I'd gotten from my uncle, one of the greatest Tibetan masters of this art. And so when I washed the dress I always had that on, and the shawl around my top—just in case the Sergeant came out. Long-Life was getting more and more filthy, tormented by the fleas and lack of any freedom to move—although he never complained. I spent a lot of time making up different impossible schemes to help him.

That week when I went to see the Captain he was really coming along quite well, considering how new he was to yoga. He went through the series I'd given him, careful this time to do things the right way—even if it was a little slower, or he couldn't get all the way into something. I let him go to the end in peace, because sometimes a student needs that too. After he had rested and let his body warm down, he sat up and looked at me with a big smile.

"I'm getting much better, aren't I?"

"Oh yes, yes, you are. And we can both see it. I want to thank you for working so well, so consistently—a little each day. I know your back is coming along, and I know the other two can see it too."

"And so you have nothing to complain about today? Nothing to make up a quotation from the Master about?"

"I don't make them up. And I think you know that by now."

He gazed at me thoughtfully. "Perhaps so, perhaps not. Time will tell. And so you are saying you've memorized the whole thing?"

I nodded, then we were quiet for a while. And then just to make sure his confidence didn't slip into cockiness I added, "There was . . . there was one small thing, though."

The Captain scowled a bit, but didn't lose his good mood.

"So let's hear it."

"Everything you did, you did well. But you skipped something, you skipped the Boat Pose."

He made a face. In fact this is one pose that everybody makes a face about: it's hard to sit there, stretch out your legs, and hold your feet up in the air while your teacher goes through a very slow count.

"That one's really a pain," he said. "I start puffing and my stomach feels like someone's walking on it—I think it's just something about me, about the way my particular body's built. I'm sure other people find it helpful, and easier to do. But it's certainly not for me. So I've just decided to leave it out. Anyway, it saves some time, and I've certainly got enough to work on with all those other poses."

"Not the point, Captain. The poses I give you have a special order, and a special purpose to the order. Each pose balances every other pose, and the effect on you and your back flows in a certain way, building towards a certain goal. When you leave even just one pose out you disrupt that flow, and you hurt that goal, in ways you cannot even realize."

He held his eyes on me. He really was improving, in the most important way: in his attitude. No petulant objections this time. And so I knew I could take him a little deeper.

"And the Master says . . ."

"Ah! The Master says! I knew it!" But he said it with a smile.

I smiled back a bit too. "The Master says, in his *Short Book:*

> *And there will come a time*
> *When differences no longer harass you.*
> II.48"

"Differences?" he said

"Differences," I repeated. "But differences first of all in the sense of preferences. As you get further and further along with your yoga, especially as the channels begin to open, and the inner winds can flow better . . ."

"Channels again. Inner winds again."

"Later," I said again. "So as you get further, and deep inside you energy begins to flow better, then things begin to tend towards unity, and less towards difference."

"Things? What kinds of things?"

"*Everything*, actually," I replied. "But right now we're talking about the poses, and fixing your back. And you can get to that further faster if you try to tone down your preferences, try to bring the differences between the poses closer together. That does a lot for your inner winds, and that does a lot for your back, and I really do promise I'll explain all of that for you very soon.

"So right now you have to attack your whole routine of poses with the same enthusiasm, with the same joy about why you're doing them, all of them. It's all for . . ."

"For a drunken wreck and a die-hard lazybones, I know." He was joking, but then I knew he was really keeping the others in mind, and my heart leaped. If he kept that up, this whole thing might work out after all.

I nodded. "Right. So you see, no pose is less important than another — some are easier for you, some are harder; everyone's different that way — but you have to come to each one with an open heart, knowing it brings you a little closer towards helping those other people we talked about. And this again is why your yoga will only succeed if you do it for something bigger than yourself.

"So no more faces when you come to a pose that's hard for you. The hard ones are usually doing you and your back the most good. Don't give in to preferences; don't create more differences in your life. It's the differences that harass us all day long, that make our days unhappy. I like this, I don't like that. I like her, I don't like him. I don't want to do this thing I have to do, I'd rather do that other thing I want to do."

We paused there and he nodded like a good soldier—almost bowed his head at me, I thought; but then the Sergeant with his sickly breath was pulling me back by the arm to my cell. I chanced a peek at my neighbor Busuku, whom I'd never really seen. He was there, sitting in a corner—a short man with a broad bald head and a cheerful belly. He gave me a bold happy wink as we passed.

7

Cultivating the Practice

First Week of April

The Captain walked in the front door with a dark look on his face, went to his room, and slammed the door. It began to feel like one of those days when things went wrong. Maybe it was the moon. Maybe it was something deeper than that. He called for me immediately.

"Little snaps won't hurt! Little pops are fine! It's all normal! Well now you've done it! My back hurts so bad I can hardly move!"

I stepped behind him and poked him here and there, and watched him twitch and jump. I could almost feel the winds jammed up in a ball at the bottom of his back. He really had hurt himself.

"How did you do this?" I asked.

"How did I do it?" he looked at me incredulously. "I did it doing your yoga, of course!"

But something in his tone said otherwise. "Oh, I see, you did it practicing your poses. Which pose were you on when it happened?"

"The one where you sit down and turn around to look behind you," he said.

"A back twist, I see. And what breath were you on when you did it?" I'd been very clear he should only hold that for two or three breaths.

"Number eight," he said proudly.

"Number eight? I told you to stop after two or three."

"Yes, I know, but ... you see ... I'm not like your average student, you see. I'm quite a determined person. And so on some of the poses I've doubled or tripled the number of breaths that I hold them. I figure it will heal my back twice as fast, you see."

I smiled at him, but felt sorry for his back. "It doesn't work that way, Captain ..."

"The Master says," he intoned, rolling his eyes.

"Yes, that's right. The Master says,

You must cultivate your practice,
Over an extended period of time.
I.14A

You can't rush it, you see. Fixing your back is not like fixing a broken chair—just pop in a new piece and sit on it. It's more like straightening out a young tree that's been growing a little crooked.

"Let me ask you something. How long have you been bending over this desk here?"

"I received my commission as Captain of this facility over ten years ago," he declared with a flourish.

"I thought so. And so your back has been slouched over, slowly jamming itself into itself, for thousands and thousands of days—do you see?"

He nodded glumly; he knew where this was going.

"And you can't just push it back straight in a few weeks; you have to go slowly, very gradually, or you might hurt it, the way you would hurt a tree if you didn't cultivate it— if you didn't coax it back to straightness, slowly, steadily, patiently."

"How slow?" he demanded, with exasperation.

"Not the thousands of days it took to ruin your back, but not just a few dozen days either." I pointed to some of the dust-laden stacks of paper off behind the mat where the Captain sat to do his work. "Can we use some of these stacks of paper for a while? Do you refer to them often?"

"Often?" he chuckled. "Never. Copies of my old reports to the Superintendent, off in the capital. The lies I get paid for . . . " He stared for a moment at the ground.

I didn't ask. I went and took a pile of papers about three inches high off of one stack, and came and set it down at his feet.

"Now we shouldn't just stop. Your back will tighten up worse than ever and it will be a real chore to work it out again. So gently now—we'll just do a little these next two weeks or so. Start with the Strong Stretch Pose: lean down, but don't touch your fingers to your toes. Touch the top sheet of paper instead."

He did. "Hold there for five breaths," I said, and he did that too. Then he straightened up, and I took just a single sheet of paper off the top of the stack, returning it to the large pile.

"One paper a day," I said. "That's the right speed for your back."

"But there must be several hundred sheets of paper there!" he exclaimed. "It will take me months to reach the floor."

"Don't think of it like that," I said. "Think of how fast it is compared to the years it took you to hurt your back in the first place."

There was a long pause; the Captain was coming around to a certain thought, rather slowly actually, but I let him come. It was amazing to consider that Katrin had put up with the same things during my own student days.

"So there's . . . there's no faster way?" he stumbled. "I mean . . . one that won't cause me any problems, of course."

I gazed towards the window as if to mull his question over. It doesn't help with certain students if they realize that you're miles ahead of them.

"There is a faster way," I said finally. "Although . . . *faster* is hardly the word. It would be more accurate to call it the *certain* way: the way that always works. And it happens to work a lot faster than the other way—the way that only works sometimes, and that only when this one does."

He looked a little confused.

"Let's just say that, if you are really serious, then I will show you how yoga really works. And if you learn how yoga really works and *then* do your yoga, well then your back will be sure to heal, the fastest way there is."

"I'm serious," he said, with a hand to his back and—thankfully—a glance at the door, and the world of the two men beyond it.

"We're agreed then," I said. "Next class we'll go into the channels, and the inner winds." I showed him how to take care of himself in the meantime, and then I was back to my cell.

When important things are about to happen, bigger problems come to try to stop them. This is a law of yoga, and a law of the powers that run our lives. A boy came in that day with Busuku's tray; the Sergeant was occupied in one of the side rooms, and so the cup came over. I gulped down a part, poured the rest into my hand, and slid the cup back. I turned to put my hand through the hole to my dear little companion, when I heard a scuff of feet behind me. I froze.

"Girl, come here." It was the Sergeant. It was the first time really he had ever spoken to me in my cell.

I closed my hand around the precious little grains of rice, and came up towards the front. He was already inside my door, his face tight with tension and his fingers working on the stick.

"Show me your hand."

I held it out.

"Open it."

I opened it. Little pieces of rice fell off the edge of my palm, in slow motion. And then there was a blur and I looked at my arm and there was a long red welt there, and slowly a line of skin separated down the middle of it, and blood began to ooze out.

"Just so you know what it feels like," said the Sergeant, and he wheeled around out the door, barring it back in a flash. And then the pain hit me and I dropped on my knees to the floor, and then there was the sound of a struggle next door, and then the steady *whoosh, whoosh* of the stick, and Busuku screaming and screaming and the Sergeant gasping for breath and finally just the silence.

φ

A little after dark that night the Sergeant went outside. I waited a long time and then whispered, "Busuku . . . Busuku . . . are you there? Are you all right?"

I heard him get up with a little groan and shuffle over to the front corner.

"Not as bad as I could be," he said slowly. "There's a skill to it, you see. You get yourself into a corner, so they can't get a full swing, you see. You got to cover up your head, and your face. And then you scream like hell, so they think they're doing some real damage, you see, and that calms them down after a bit." He paused. "But now we really have to talk."

"Oh yes, I'm so sorry. I didn't think . . . "

"It's all right," he said. "But you've got to know how it goes, now. The Sergeant within a day of course knew I was giving you food."

"Well how do people get their own food around here?"

"They don't," he chuckled. "This is the old-style jail: your family or friends bring you food, or else you starve to death, and they just throw your body out on the road there. Why would someone like the Sergeant want to give somebody like you or me a free ride?"

"And so those boys who come—they . . . they are your family?"

"Family?" he chuckled again. "Well yes, I guess you could say family, in a way. They work for me."

"Work for you?"

"Well for us, actually. For the good Sergeant and me."

"You and the Sergeant? You work together? Are you some kind of . . . some kind of government officer then?"

He laughed, and then caught himself. "Oh no, the other way around. That would be . . . you see . . . to say that the Sergeant is a thief, and we steal things together, or used to—until we got in a bit of a disagreement, like all thieves do. How to split the stuff up, you see, and me with all the boys to feed."

"But where are their families; what about their parents?"

"No families, no parents. All orphans. Parents dead, parents gone, parents that didn't want them. And so I take them in, and I teach them."

"Teach them . . . to steal?"

"Keeps them fed," he replied in a hurt tone. Then he added quickly, "And we've got to figure out how to keep you fed too. Now people without anyone to bring them food can just buy their food from the Sergeant, for about ten times what it really costs . . . "

"But I have no money."

"Figured that much," he said again, speaking quickly. "Then the only other option is if they'll let you do some kind of work. I figure that's what the Sergeant has in mind, and that's why he decided to force the issue today, and then stepped out so we'd end up talking about it."

"Oh, I wouldn't mind to work—I did a lot of work growing up."

"Whatever work the Sergeant has in mind may not be what you expect. Be careful with him. Try to bring it up with the Captain first."

"But I won't see him for another week now." And then there was a noise at the front porch.

"Remember to look hungry," Busuku whispered cryptically, and the Sergeant was back.

8

Channels of Light

Second Week of April

Katrin and my travels had taught me to go without food for days at a time and not even notice it much, but a week I knew would leave me very weak, and I was afraid for Long-Life. There didn't seem to be much choice though, and so I settled down for the siege and tried to ignore the smell of Busuku's daily tray.

The second night, very late, I woke suddenly. Long-Life was growling—the first time in all these weeks that he'd made any noise at all. And then I heard something drop, and the sound of little feet running away. A few minutes later there was a faint snuffle at the hole; I crawled over silently and looked.

Long-Life was using his nose to push through a little package wrapped in fresh green leaves. Inside was a cake of rice, with raisins and nuts. We gulped it down, and I pushed the leaves out into the trench behind the wall. It went like that every night then, and during the day I was careful to lie listless on the floor of my cell. The Sergeant was waiting, and watching.

The week went by and I tried to shuffle along slowly when the Sergeant took me to see the Captain.

"Your back—is it better?" I asked.

"Much better; feels like it will be back to where it was before, in another week or so."

I came around and touched the spot. Things were much looser—the winds were breaking up and starting to flow again. I stepped back in front, told him I thought he was probably right, and pointed to the center of the room. "Good then, let's see your routine—the *patient* version please," I smiled.

But his eyes were glued on my arm. The cut was long and ugly now—I didn't have enough extra water to keep it clean, and no matter how I tried to cover it with a corner of my dress, the flies were getting into it.

"The Sergeant . . . had to discipline you for something?"

"For trying to eat," I smiled, but inside I was ready to burst out crying. "Captain, sir, if there is any honest work I could do, for some food . . . "

He waved his hand and cut me off. "Talk to the Sergeant. The Sergeant runs the jail part."

"But . . . but you are the Captain. You run the whole place."

"That's correct. I'm the Captain, and I run the entire station. And he's the Sergeant, and he runs the jail. Talk to the Sergeant."

"But the jail is *part* of the station."

"That's correct," he said, skating ahead with official logic. "And it's the part that the Sergeant is in charge of." He gave me an odd look, as though I were especially stupid and couldn't grasp what he was saying. "Talk to the Sergeant," he repeated, and walked over to start his poses.

When he was done I took out a few poses that I was still afraid he might overdo, and added some at the end which would loosen up his back more, before he got up to continue his day. Then I had him stand before me.

"Captain, have you ever known anyone who tried to learn yoga?"

He gave me a strange look, then turned his eyes to the window. "I have," he replied, "or you wouldn't be here now."

I looked the question at him.

"The Sergeant would have shipped you off to the prison, the one in the capital," he said, "for theft of valuable property. No one who didn't know something about yoga would have ever believed you—being a girl, and all."

I looked down at the floor bitterly. It was true, as I had learned long ago, even back in my own country. I collected myself, and avoided the obvious questions. Where had he seen yoga? And did *he* believe me now? It would come, in time.

"Then you probably know," I said, "that many people *try* yoga. For a good number of them yoga works wonderfully: it helps them recover their strength and energy, fixes problems like your back, makes them look slender, bright, and happy.

"Other people try yoga, and it seems to work fairly well for them, if not as amazing as with the others. And still other people try but can't seem to pick it up very well; or yoga just seems boring, or a chore; or they're simply too busy, and they drop it. A few people even have a bad experience with it."

The Captain nodded. "I have seen all those types." He didn't seem ready to say more, but my curiosity was piqued. How much did he know, from before?

"And so did you ever wonder, why yoga seems to work for some people, but not for others?"

He shrugged, as if it didn't strike him as very important. "I don't know, everyone's different. Some people try it and take to it, some people try it and don't."

"But they *try* it," I said. "That's the point, you see. They *try* it, because they think it might help them—help them feel better, help them look better. And then it works for some of them, and it doesn't work for others. Didn't you ever wonder why?"

He shrugged again, looking a little bored.

"But it's important, you see. Yoga is a pretty serious thing to start. It takes a good amount of effort and it takes a good amount of time. And in many cases people try it for some very serious reasons—they've hurt themselves somehow, or they need to make a big change in their lives. And so they try. But why try, and try so hard, if you can't be sure it's going to work for you?"

This caught his attention—it dawned on him that we were also talking about whether or not yoga would work for *him*.

"I see your point," he said, with more thought now, "but I don't see where you're going. Yoga just works for some people, and doesn't work for others. You just have to try and find out which type you are. That's just the way it is."

I shook my head with a violence that threw my long black hair whipping across my face. His eyes left to it for a moment, but then snapped back, as if there were something he didn't want to think about. "*Just the way it is* doesn't exist. 'Just the way it is' is a lie. And it's a lie that people use to cover up the fact that they won't take the time or the trouble to figure out how things really work.

"Now yoga works. It works for the people that it works for, although it seems like most of the time they don't exactly know *why* it worked for them: they just don't think about it. Then maybe at some point—later on, when they get older, say—it stops working for them, and they're stuck.

"And yoga would also work for the ones that it doesn't seem to work for; they just need someone to teach them *how* it works. It's a terrible thing to think of someone going around for the rest of their life with something that hurts as much as your back does, just because no one ever showed them first *how* yoga works. You see the idea?"

With that he gave a good Captain's nod. He sensed a plan of action.

"So I'm going to start teaching you *how* yoga works; because if you know *that*, then it will *always* work for you. And there are . . . "

" . . . two other people's lives at stake, at least," filled in the Captain thoughtfully, and I wanted to hug him. He was really on the right track.

"Exactly. And so we'll keep going with the poses, but now we'll spend a little time each class talking about *how* they work, to make sure they *do* work.

"And everything I tell you about how yoga works will come from the Master's *Short Book,* because that's really what it's all about. It makes sense that that's what it *would* be about: the reason his book has been around for so many centuries is that it's so very clear about how yoga really works, you see?"

The Captain nodded happily, his mission and his orders both put before him so solidly.

"Now turn around and take off your shirt," I ordered him. My own Teacher, Katrin, had had this warm but very formal way of touching me when it was really needed—to correct something, or to show me how something flowed in me under the skin—and I was careful to set the same tone now with the Captain.

"From here," I said, touching the top of his head, "down to here." And I gently nudged his back, near his waist. "This is the part that the Master is talking about when he says,

Turn the combined effort
Upon the sun,
And you will understand
The earth.

III.27"

"Combined effort . . . of what and what?" he asked, without turning around.

"Later," I admonished. Then I ran the tip of my finger slowly down the length of his back, just off to the right side of the middle, between the same two points on his head and his spine.

"Under here is a channel nicknamed the 'sun,'" I said.

"Channel?" he asked. "You mean like a muscle, or a nerve?"

"No, neither one of those, although you can picture it looking like a nerve if it helps you. But really it's much finer than that—very fine and subtle, as if it were made of light itself; not something you'd ever be able to see if you cut someone open.

"And you have lots of channels like that—running all through your body. They begin to grow even before the rest of you does, inside your mother's womb—a whole network of extremely subtle tubes, branching out. And in fact the nerves and the blood vessels and even the bones and flesh form then around these channels, like ice around the branches and twigs of a tree, so that the entire structure of our bodies is really a perfect reflection of this network of luminous channels.

"Now it so happens that all of this starts from here," I continued, pressing the tip of my finger lightly into his back, right where he had his problem. "The network begins growing, inside your mother, from this point along the back, right behind your belly button. That's why the Master says,

> *Turn the same effort*
> *Upon the center at the navel,*
> *And you will understand*
> *The structure of the body.*
>
> III.30"

"What does he mean by 'center'?" asked the Captain, still facing the other way, but obviously very interested.

"It's an image of a wheel—of like a wagon wheel, with spokes," I said. "In the ancient Mother Tongue, in Sanskrit, they call it a *chakra*. As this network of subtle channels begins to grow, they branch off like spokes of a wheel, off to the sides, from this point at your back. And then other channels, including the biggest and most important ones, begin to branch off up and down—and your spine for example grows along their pattern.

"So if you had very specially tuned eyes, and you could see the channels, then if you looked straight down someone's spine you could see channels branching out, like spokes of a wheel, from special points or centers along the back."

"And so the channel called the 'sun' runs inside me, up and down, where you drew the line with your finger? And it's one of the more important channels?"

"That's right," I said—so glad that he was listening carefully. It would help so much to fix his back. "And that's why the Master mentions it first."

"But when you say 'channel' or 'tube'" the Captain thought out loud, "you seem to be saying that they are hollow—and that perhaps something flows inside of them."

"Exactly right," I said, "and I'll tell you more about that later. Right now let's just say that one of the things running back and forth in these channels is thought itself: your own thoughts are flowing along this network of tubes made of stuff as fine as sunlight.

"Now if you think about it," I went on, "you could take all the things we ever think about and divide them into two types. The first type would be, well, just things—things like the wall over there, or your desk, or even your back, where it hurts." I poked his back again, a little harder, to keep his mind there with me. He winced nicely and I went on.

"And then there's thinking itself—your own mind. We can hear ourselves think, we can be aware of our thoughts. And so everything we ever think about is either objects like the wall, or the mind itself."

He nodded, but I could see he was getting a little tired, especially after all the poses. Time to tie all this down to how yoga really was going to work for his back.

"Now the thoughts that run along this sun channel," and I ran my finger again down the right side of his spine, "they're the ones that concentrate on the more concrete side of things, you see. Things that are more solid, like solid earth. And that's why the Master says you can understand the 'earth' if you understand this channel. He means you can understand how the thoughts that run in this channel see the objects in the world around us. And then you can fix your back."

"Fix my back? How's that? What's the connection?"

"It's this," I said, "and then we'll stop—it's too much to tell you in one day. You see, the thoughts that run in this sun channel along your back, they are wrong thoughts. They are mistaken thoughts. They don't see things right at all.

"And that causes a disturbance in the channel, you see, and that causes a block in the center that we spoke about, right here," I poked his back again so he'd remember all this.

"And that's what makes my back hurt," he breathed.

"And that's what makes your back hurt," I repeated. "That's *really* what makes your back hurt."

"Fix that and fix my back?"

"Fix that and fix your back, fix anyone's back."

He turned and began to button his shirt. And he glanced down at his desk. "It's not such a small book after all," he mused.

φ

"Sergeant, sir," I turned to him as he opened the door to my cell. He looked down at me with those red eyes, like a cat who's cornered a mouse. "I need food; I have to eat. I don't have family here, I don't have money. But I can work; I know how to work hard, if you would just let me try, I don't care how difficult it is—any . . . any honest work I can do."

He gave me a long relaxed smile; the first I had ever seen from him, and it was truly rather frightening. I could feel Busuku, in the next cell, straining to hear and to help.

"What do you know how to do, girl? What kind of skills would . . . would a *girl* have?" Another disgusting smile.

I thought of the class I'd just finished with the Captain. "I know yoga," I said. "I can teach yoga, and I can also teach the Mother Tongue—our ancient books of Sanskrit."

The Sergeant let out a crude guffaw. "I said a *skill*, girl! You know, something somebody would be willing to *pay* you for."

I blushed and looked at the floor. The most precious things in the world have no value to the world. And then I remembered something else.

"I can weave," I said. "I am a very good weaver, and a fast one."

The Sergeant paused, staring down at me, calculating. Then he yelled out, "Busuku!"

"Why yes . . . *Sir!*" came an ironic voice, from behind the other wall.

"If you want to sneak a few cups of old rice to this idiot girl, please feel free to do so. If she can't weave like she says she can, or perform some other . . . *useful* service, shall we say . . . then she won't be with us much longer anyway."

"Yes, . . . *Sir,*" came the voice again—mocking, but just a little less than would warrant the stick, and we all knew it.

9

North Star

Third Week of April

The nighttime packages through the back hole stopped, and rather generous cups of rice and beans, and even some tasty little surprises, began again from the front corner. I noticed that these little extras—say a handful of peanuts—always appeared when the corporal was on duty. And then he'd sit, slumped there on the bench with his little pot belly sticking out, and go through a huge pile of peanuts himself as he stared at the ceiling or the opposite wall. Cracking them open, one by one, and dropping the shells listlessly to the floor, into the little piles of dirt and rubbish already there, for who knows how long.

"What are these?" asked the Captain at our next class. He held out the pieces of parchment that I always kept wrapped at the back of the *Short Book*.

I reached out unconsciously and touched them with reverence—just the touch was so reassuring. "Those are the notes—the notes I took in my own language, in Tibetan, when my Teacher taught me the *Short Book about Yoga*. And the translation we made of it is there as well. They are absolutely priceless, more so even than the Master's book here, since other copies of it can still be found."

The Captain nodded thoughtfully, and placed the pages back with care.

"Do you still believe I stole this book—that I *could* steal such a book?" I asked, point-blank.

He looked at me for a moment, and then glanced down. "That is still . . . under investigation," he said.

"Investigation? Investigation by whom?"

"By the Sergeant," he replied bluntly, and my face fell. "The Sergeant has been conducting this investigation, to see if anyone is missing the book."

"Investigation?" I repeated. "Anyone? How many people around here would ever own a book like this? Could even read it?"

The Captain appraised me sternly. "Perhaps . . . perhaps more than you might think," he said slowly. And he closed the cloth over the book softly, and we began our lesson.

His back was nearly returned to its normal painful level, and I realized that at this point what he needed was not more poses, but to go deeper into the ones he already had—to hold them deeper than before. This is one of the most difficult things for anyone to practice outside of their classes with their teacher, and I reminded him again to keep his mission in mind whenever it seemed difficult to go deeper: "The other two are watching. The other two need to be healed too. You have to be steady, and you have to be willing to *work*."

He was gleaming in a fine sweat by the time he laid down for his rest at the end. Inside, I smiled. He already looked so much better, and he didn't really realize it. "Just like all students," I sighed to myself.

I stood him up again facing the wall behind his desk, and traced a line with my finger again from the tip of his head to the same point on his spine. But this time I drew it just slightly off to the left of the center of his back.

"The channel that we call the 'sun' has a twin. And here the Master says,

> *You will understand*
> *The arrangement of the stars*
> *If you turn this same effort*
> *Upon the moon.*
>
> II.28

So as you would guess, the name we give to the twin is the 'moon' channel."

"Why the 'sun' and the 'moon'?" broke in the Captain. "Do these channels have anything to do with the real sun and moon?"

I saw Katrin clearly in my mind, bending over the tunnels the mole had made in the garden, trying to explain it to me.

"It's not something we should go into right now," I said. But to plant a seed for later I added, "If more and more layers of ice pile up on a branch, it gets a little harder to tell how each bump reflects a smaller one on the branch itself."

There was a pause, and the Captain's pride—that man thing, you know—kept him from asking what he wanted to. "I see," he said with assurance. "Please go on."

"Now as you might also guess, this other channel is where your thoughts about the other half of things flow— not thoughts about concrete objects and stuff like that, you see, but thoughts about your own thoughts: thoughts about your own mind, you see—about the fact that we can think or sense things at all.

"So for example you could say that when you think about your bad back, that thought is running in the sun channel. But when you think about how it *feels*, when you think about your awareness of the pain, well then that thought is running in this channel, in the moon channel. Got it?"

"Got it," he replied. "Bad back thought in the channel on the right side. Ouch thought in the channel on the left side."

I nodded and smiled. He was really getting the hang of all of this rather well, all the way from the poses on up to the ideas about how the poses really worked. And I knew this would be the thing to heal him.

"Now if the things in the world around us are like the earth, then our thoughts—and all the different parts of our minds—are like the stars: tiny points of light, tiny sparks of awareness scattered throughout our bodies. And the most important ones relate to the centers we spoke about: crucial junctures of branch channels along the length of the back— along the most important channel of all. This channel the Master describes in these lines:

> *Turn the effort*
> *Upon the polestar,*
> *And you will understand*
> *Their movement.*
>
> III.29"

Now I used my knuckle and ran a line straight down the middle of the Captain's back, from the top of his head to that point at his waist, right behind his belly button. "This is the middle channel, running down the body as its core, as the axis from which all the other channels branch out. And so it's like the North Star—the polestar—sitting on top of that great invisible axis around which all the other stars turn, during the course of the night.

"It's only because of this immobile axis that we can see the motion of the stars, and it's only because of this middle channel that we can understand how the stars in our own body—our own thoughts and sparks of awareness—run within their channels. For this is the channel of understanding itself: this middle one is where the good thoughts flow— thoughts of purity, and goodness; thoughts of peace and wisdom."

I held my finger there for a moment where his back hurt and pictured the middle channel opening up again to where it had once been, and then even further, forever further.

10

Horses and Horsemen

Fourth Week of April

"Sit down," said the Captain, at the very start of our next class together. "I have some good news for you."

My heart leapt; surely he had decided that the book was my own, and that I was free to go. And then another thought came upon the first: my job was not yet finished, neither with the Captain, nor with those other two unhappy souls. But I was saved the decision.

"The Sergeant tells me that you have requested work," he began, and I ran my fingers ruefully over the crusted cut on my arm.

"That's true," I replied. "As per your suggestion, sir."

"Well I am happy to inform you that the Sergeant has made an arrangement with a woman who lives in a small cluster of homes out a little west of here." The Captain waved towards the back of the jail.

"You will do weaving for the woman; whatever amount she asks for. She will pay the Sergeant. The Sergeant will reimburse the woman for your food and lodging."

A little sigh of joy escaped my lips. "Lodging, sir? Am I to stay . . . to stay with the woman?"

"That's correct," smiled the Captain. "And I must say that the Sergeant is being most generous. After considerable thought, I have approved the arrangement; for two reasons, really."

I raised my eyebrows.

"First of all, I have the book, and what you say are your priceless notes. Whatever they are, I have a feeling that they are valuable, and you will not easily leave them behind."

I nodded. All too true. I had sworn to Katrin that I would make the translation and the notes into a finished book for others; to complete this task was one of the reasons I lived at all, and so it was worth even my life.

"Now secondly, there is something you should understand," he continued. "If you try to escape, you will be caught. Whatever you might think of the three of us here, you must realize that the agents of the King—his personal network, throughout the realm—are ruthless and efficient, especially with escaped prisoners. You would end up back here, or worse, but now guilty of a very serious crime, worth years in this little hole—whether it turns out that the book was yours or not. Do I make myself clear?"

Something twitched inside my stomach. Something about the Sergeant—something out of balance in what the Captain was proposing. But I realized too that I was a prisoner, and being a prisoner means not having any choices—or not realizing that you do, anyway. And so I nodded, and it was done.

"You will report to the station once each morning, and stay long enough to see whether or not I require your services," he added.

I nodded again, and he stood for his class. This time I had him turn around and remove his shirt before we began the poses.

"You need to know a little more about how the channels work," I said, "especially the three main ones: the sun, the moon, and the axis around which everything else revolves." I traced the lines this time with three fingers at once. "Then you'll really understand what the poses are doing for your back—a big part of how yoga really works."

He stood there at attention, still facing the back wall—I think he liked this part, just listening without having to relate to me face-to-face, quietly drawing pictures in his mind of the channels as I described them.

"Now we said that thoughts are running through these main three channels . . . " I began.

"Bad thoughts about things running on the right, bad thoughts about thought itself running on the left, and good thoughts up and down the middle channel," he intoned.

He'd been thinking about it at home, which would make today's lesson that much easier. Katrin had insisted that I mentally review every class three times before the next one, and I considered this method one of the greatest teachings of our ancient lineage.

"Captain, sir!" The corporal burst in the door and stopped short at his shirtless superior.

"Corporal! What are you doing! When will you learn to knock?"

"Sir! A disturbance! We . . . you must come, now!"

The Captain began pulling on his shirt. "Where is it?" he demanded.

"Why, just outside the front yard, sir! On the road there, sir!"

The Captain reached for his own stick, which was leaned up in the back corner, collecting dust.

"Will we need help?" he gasped. "How many people involved?"

"Why, no people, sir!"

61

"No people?" The Captain paused, one hand on his stick and the other on his bad back.

"Why no, sir, only a cow, sir!"

"A cow?"

"A cow, sir! Eating up the last little bit of the hedge out front, sir!"

I pictured the front yard of the station—a flat ugly piece of dirt, devoid of anything green at all. If there had ever been a hedge, I hadn't noticed it coming in.

The Captain twirled his stick expertly in one swift gesture, like a baton. Coming around again the tip of it beaned the corporal neatly on the top of the head. It was nothing like a blow from the Sergeant—just a day's bump, I'd say.

"Corporal."

"Yes sir," cried the young man in a high voice, rubbing his nascent knot.

"Go out to that cow, yourself."

"Myself? Yes sir, myself, sir!"

"Get behind it."

"Behind it! Myself! Yes, sir!"

"Hold up its tail, rather high."

"Sir!"

"And then pull the tail, hard."

"Sir! Yes . . . *sir!*"

"And then see whether the cow poops on you, or just kicks you and breaks your leg."

"Poop? Kick? Sir?"

The Captain took the corporal strongly by the shoulders, thrust him outside, and slammed the door.

"Idiot!" he exclaimed. He turned halfway around and threw his stick into the corner, grunting and holding his back as he did.

"Sorry for the interruption," he wheezed.

"No interruption at all," I said. I suddenly remembered how Katrin had turned anything that ever happened around us into a part of the class, seamlessly. "Captain, hold out your hands, palms down."

He did so. Each hand was shaking like a leaf.

"Wonderful!" I beamed. "The contents of the channels, right there in front of us!"

He clenched his hands and put them down at his sides. "What are you talking about?" he exclaimed. "Two corporals in one day is more than any man should have to bear!"

I laughed. "Not nonsense," I said. "It's about the other thing that runs inside the channels: the inner winds."

"Winds?" he said.

"We call them winds, because—to most people at least—they are invisible like the wind; and also because they flow to and fro within the channels, together with your thoughts. And so here inside the channels is that mysterious ground where body and mind meet: the body, solid flesh and bone and blood; and the mind, invisible, untouchable, luminous with knowing, beyond all physical matter.

"Here in the channels is where the two are ultimately joined. The winds, a very subtle form of physical stuff, are like moving horses. And riding upon these winds, like a horseman upon a horse, is the mind, our thoughts. And so they always flow together, always connected, and this is what the Master is speaking of when he says,

> *The mind flies off,*
> *And with that come*
> *Pain in the body;*
> *Unhappy thoughts;*
> *Shaking in the hands*

And other parts of your body;
The breath falling out of rhythm
As it passes in and out.

I.31

And so it's like trying to concentrate on a yoga class, you see, and then some . . ." here I almost repeated the Captain's "idiot," but caught myself ". . . person interrupts you, and your mind flies off, it gets disturbed. And because of the connection between the rider and the horse—between the thoughts and the winds, inside the channels—then the winds get disturbed too, and that triggers a reaction all through your gross physical body, because the channels and the winds reach to every corner of it.

"And so the hands start to shake, reflecting the winds inside. The breath changes too, falling out of rhythm, because the one part of the body that's really tied very tightly to the winds is the breath.

"The interruption, the disturbance of our thoughts, builds up over a few minutes—or even hours and days and months, if we can't stop thinking about it, and then a kind of unhappiness sets in. And this unhappy state of mind has to be flowing in . . . " I paused to see if the Captain would complete the thought. This was a trick that Katrin had used constantly in my own classes, to make sure I was listening, and to keep me thinking.

" . . . has to be flowing in the two channels running up the back, along either side of the middle channel," finished the Captain, proud of his answer as any child in a school, and rightfully so. "Because unhappiness is a *bad* thought, you see," he added for good measure.

"Exactly," I returned. "Now there's one more thing I need to show you, and then you'll have the whole picture."

I turned him around, and had him slip his shirt off once more. Then I used the first finger of both hands to draw the side channels, sun and moon, down his back again. At several points on his back—at the bottom of his neck, right behind his heart, and again down at the point at his waist where it hurt—I crossed the lines over each other, and then back again.

"Those two bad guys—the two side channels—they go up and down the back like vines, you see. They twist at a number of points all the way around the good guy—around the middle channel—and then continue on their way. And at the points where they twist around, crossing each other, they are in a position to choke the middle channel."

"In a position to choke it?" asked the Captain.

"Right—in a position to choke it—because they can only really choke it if they are thick and strong; when . . . " I paused.

"When they are chock full of bad thoughts?" the Captain tried.

"Right again," I beamed at his back, and it straightened a touch more. "Because the thoughts and the winds they ride upon, within these three channels, you see, they're like air pumped into one of those long goatskin balloons that children play with. Squeeze the air out of one side—say the good side—and it goes over and makes the bad side fatter. Except that in this case, the bad side is also wrapped around the good side, which makes it even harder to get the air back to the good side."

"So what you're saying here is that—when I get upset at the corporal, say—the thoughts are running so strong and hard in my side channels that they close in at certain places on the middle channel, which makes it even more difficult for me to get un-upset."

"Just so," I agreed. "Now, last thing before we get you on to the poses. Do you remember where the lines on your back crisscrossed?"

"Neck, middle of the back, and lower back—right where mine is hurt."

I held my breath and let him come to it on his own.

"The places . . . " he said, with growing excitement " . . . the exact places where people most often hurt themselves—and where people as they get older start to freeze up, with arthritis and the like."

"Exactly," I said. "Keep up a line of negative thoughts long enough, choke the middle channel hard enough, often enough, and you start having what the Master calls 'pain in the body,' you see, in exactly those places . . . "

"And the poses then," he rushed on. "The poses—each one must do something to loosen up those choke points, to get the winds back flowing again in the middle channel.

"Which would also make you have more of the right thoughts," he added thoughtfully, "the good ones—the ones that flow there, in the middle channel."

I turned him around and gave him a big sunny smile. "I guess that's why you're the Captain," I said, and then took him through a good hard routine so he wouldn't get a big head.

11

Breath and
a Smile

First Week of May

The next day the Sergeant came rather unceremoniously, opened the door to my cell, and waved his stick towards the front door of the station. I gathered up my bag with the shawl and bowl and said, for Busuku's sake, "So I am to go for my work, at the weaver's?"

The Sergeant didn't react at all—just to let me know that he knew by now everything that ever went on between prisoners. He tapped his stick on the floor, but actually looked as relaxed as I'd ever seen him, in an expectant sort of way; and that in itself got me nervous in my stomach again.

Going past the Captain's open door I peeked to the side, and caught him peeking too. I nodded in a way that said he didn't need to worry about having trusted me. And he really didn't. I don't know what age it is when you figure it out—I suppose with some people it must be later than sooner—but I had already come to realize that whether I was happy or not had just about nothing to do with the kind of place I was staying in.

And here at the jail I had a captive audience, you see:
I had at least one person who would stick with what I
was teaching him because he was hurting, and it would
make him better. And oh how glorious it would be then if,
together, we could heal the other two broken souls. They
say that the most stunning flower of all—the lotus—grows
in the filthiest part of the pond, feeds on the filth to produce
its beauty. And so stepping out of the jail didn't feel much
different to me really than sitting inside of it. It was fertile
ground for what I had to give.

On the porch I turned and touched the Sergeant warmly
on the arm. He jumped and stared at me; I stepped away to
the side, smoothly, with a little wave, the way Grandmother
would have done.

"I'll be right back," I said breezily. "Just got to get the
dog."

The Sergeant was so taken aback that he didn't think to
stop me. "On the *rope*," he called out, when I was already
halfway to the back of the building.

If you have ever lived with one of those Tibetan lap dogs,
then I don't have to tell you what my reunion with Long-
Life was like. Wild circles singing to the sky, wrapping my
legs in the rope.

"Shush now, little lion. I love you too. But the Sergeant's
a little free with his stick, and I don't think either one of us
should push our luck."

It was about a half hour's walk to the old woman's little
house. There was a rickety shed out behind, and she'd set
up a small loom there, with a pile of fresh straw this time
on the floor. She was a short stocky widow, with unkempt
white hair. Life had carved its lines deep into her face, and
she had struggled while it did.

She didn't speak to me much. On that first day, after the Sergeant left, she looked at me with a scowl, held her nose with disgust, and sent me off to a stream nearby with orders not to return until me, and my dress, and "that disgusting mongrel" were all washed and dried. The stream ran between two fields that had just been tilled and planted; they were huge and ran in either direction as far as the eye could see. I found a small wooden bridge with some bushes growing on one side, where we could sit and dry without being seen. The water and the sun were glorious, but Long-Life and I didn't tarry; I would not provide the Sergeant with any excuse to lock us up for good.

As for the work, there's not much to say. Just the usual: I wore my fingers to the bone churning out thin, shoddy little rugs that my mistress could sell quickly and easily in town on market day. Any suggestions I had for the rich designs and deep pile of the rugs we made in my homeland of Tibet were met with stony silence, and an order to get back to work.

The Sergeant came several times and stayed too long, out behind the house, listening to the woman's lies about how much food the dog and I were going through every day. He would shut the bargaining off with a tap of his stick when he got impatient, hand back the woman a few coins, and then walk straight off to town for his liquor. And every morning I was at the jail bright and early, sitting on the little bench, well before the Captain arrived.

On the day he called for his next class, I stopped him about halfway through the poses.

"It's time we talked about breathing," I said; he was in fact puffing already and seemed quite grateful to pause and listen.

"If there's anything about our outside physical body that most affects the inner winds, it's not actually the poses themselves," I said. "Our breath is even more linked to the winds. And so if we can breathe in a way that keeps the winds from causing stoppages in the channels, the poses become infinitely more effective. If on the other hand we breathe in fits and stops while we go through our poses, it can do more harm to the channels than good—causing tie-ups like the one that makes your back hurt.

"So let's go through some practical advice from the Master—tips on getting the breath to flow right, which can be a whole science in itself, even if you never do any series of poses."

The Captain nodded. I noticed he was already making an effort to get his breath flowing smoothly again, right then and there. He really had great instincts—or something—for yoga, for everything involved with yoga.

"When the Master talks about how to breathe, what he says first is:

> *Keep a close watch*
> *On the breath;*
> *Outside or inside,*
> *Stopped or being exchanged.*
>
> II.50A

Now the first and most obvious thing to say about your breathing as you go through the poses is that you should always breathe through your nose, and not through your mouth—unless of course you have some serious blockage of your nostrils. If there's a blockage that's caused by some kind of congestion—lots of mucus—then before starting your session you should do your best to clear it out. You can blow your nose, or do even more effective things that free it up—special techniques that the sages of old discovered, and that I would rather show you than tell you about, should the need arise. But you should really keep an eye on whether your nostrils and the nasal passages behind them are in any way blocked or constricted: if they are, it could really be making the poses much more difficult to do, and less effective.

"I say 'less effective' in one sense because of the connection between your nasal passages and those three main channels we are trying to work on, to loosen. These three don't just stop at the top of your head; the two side channels come down inside your skull and then out on each side of the top of your nose—this is in fact why your nose grows with two nostrils in the first place. And the middle channel comes down and ends behind a spot on the lower part of your forehead, just above the point halfway between your eyebrows. So when you breathe in and out not through your mouth but through your nose, and smoothly, it has a way of helping to calm the flow of the inner winds within the three channels, with their opening so close to the nose. This then helps loosen the choke-points around the important centers along the back and head."

The Captain was listening carefully; I knew it from the sound of his breath, which was growing softer and softer. When we listen to something intently the mind is focused, and this slows the inner winds, which slows the breath. All connected, I thought.

"Now at different points in your poses we want all the breath to be either outside your body or inside your body. This happens for example when you do that very first pose: Bowing to the Sun. At the exact point when you are reaching for the sky—at the very point when you are stretching to the limit—your breath is all inside: you are at the very end of an inhale of your breath. The stretch should be a very natural, smooth, and happy experience—like what you do naturally when you stretch your arms out in a good huge yawn: feels great. Your lungs are full, radiant with the air, and your blood is drinking in its food, the oxygen.

"There are other points when all the breath should have gone outside the body: like in the very next step of the same pose, where you bend over to touch your toes. As you reach your furthest point down, your tummy should be squeezing in and making sure every last drop of air that you can get out of the lungs is out—out to the outside, delivering the carbon dioxide waste from your blood back to the air of the world.

"If you don't get the fresh air in, full, the body won't have enough fuel. If you don't get the used air out, there's no place for the next breath of fresh air. And then the breath begins to go out of rhythm, right there, starting to move just a touch in stops and starts. This then puts a little more pressure on the middle channel, where the two side channels choke it."

"Middle channel choked," broke in the Captain, "fewer happy thoughts. And then in a few minutes you're not feeling happy doing the poses—it begins to feel like work, or even a little tense."

"Just right," I nodded. "And then the muscles tense up a bit, just a bit, and that knocks the breathing more out of balance, and that disturbs the winds in the channels rather than smoothing them out—which is what the poses are *supposed* to do—and then well eventually it's just not much fun, and you give up your yoga, along with every hope of really curing something like your bad back forever.

"Now you especially have to watch that the breathing never stops, or gets held up. There's a natural pause for a split second right between the end of one breath and the start of another, and again as the lungs reach the full point—just before you exhale. And there are other situations where the breath pauses, sometimes for quite some length of time, due to a beautiful stillness of the inner winds—but we'll get to that later. During your poses though you have to be careful never to let the breath stop. The breath should always be in motion, deep motion—all the air being exchanged, in and out. Never let the breath lock up inside; never hold it when, say, you're having trouble reaching or keeping a certain position. This puts a lot of pressure on the choke-points, and that's the last thing we want.

"One last little tip, which will always help keep your breath from locking up. Remember to keep a close watch *here*," I touched his forehead, just above the point midway between his eyebrows, "and *here* too." I put a finger at each corner of his mouth, and pushed up to form a smile.

"You must be kidding," he said, looking a little bashful.

"Not at all," I said. "Dead serious. When you let a challenging pose get the better of you, then your forehead starts to scrunch together here, between your eyebrows. This is right at the delicate place where the channels are coming out, and that little frown causes blocks in the flow; that's in fact why we frown here, and not somewhere else in our bodies."

"Again choking the middle channel, setting off a chain reaction of unhappy thoughts," observed the Captain.

"Right again," I said. "And when these go up," I pulled the corners of my own mouth into a smile, "then it loosens the end points of the two side channels, up alongside the nose . . . "

"And then smiling actually sets off a flow of nice thoughts, in the middle channel," finished the Captain.

"And so a little smile, while you're doing your poses, is one of the most important poses of all," I grinned. He grinned, and finished his poses trying to grin, and then I returned to the old woman who never grinned at all.

12

Breath and Heart

Second Week of May

Before our next lesson the Captain and I talked some more about the breath; I felt like we should, because there was such a strong connection between his breath and his inner winds, choked and hurting him at the bottom of his back.

"Now about the breath, the Master also says,

> *Observe too*
> *The place in the body,*
> *The duration, and the count.*
>
> II.50B

What he means first of all about watching the place in your body is that—as you do your poses, or other practices—you should have very conscious control about which part of your body you are using to breathe with. In most cases you get the most fresh air, most easily, if you breathe by moving your diaphragm: the big sheet of muscle that closes in the bottom of your ribcage."

The Captain looked a little uncertain. I held my hand on his chest and said, "Try to take a few breaths without making my hand move."

He fidgeted a little and then stuck his tummy way out to take a breath. I giggled a bit—but I could also see that his stomach was getting leaner, and more flat.

"Right idea; a bit off on the location," I said. "Try a little higher up—concentrate on the place just below your ribs."

He did, and it went fine. "That's best for deep breathing," I said. "It also has a way of keeping the whole area around your tummy—especially down around your waist and below that—firm and strong, as you go through your poses. Strength there has a very powerful effect on your lower back, helping it immensely in holding up your entire upper body. All this in turn prevents tie-ups at major choke-points in your lower back, all the way down through your lower organs of digestion and excretion, the reproductive organs, and the different parts of the legs themselves.

"Now there are also poses that tie up the diaphragm, and force you to send the breath to other parts of your lungs, to keep them healthy and well fed with fresh air. One pose like this is the one named after the wise man Marichi . . . "

"Where you've got your foot up against your belly and the only way you can breathe is if you *do* move your ribs," said the Captain.

"Right," I said. "Now you can also send the breath, just in your mind, to a part of your body where you're not so strong yet, to give it sort of an energy boost."

"You mean that, say, when I'm doing that Warrior of Excellence thing—trying to bend my knees with my legs wide apart—and my thighs are shaking and I feel like I'm going to flop down on my bottom, then I could pretend to send my leg a burst of power when I take a big breath in."

I smiled. It was a perfect example; I couldn't shake the feeling that he knew more about yoga than he was letting on. "Right again. And then of course a final place in your body where you can imagine sending the power of your breath is right there into the choke-point itself: for you, right into the center located at your lower back.

"You just picture the energy of the breath flowing down and freeing up the middle channel, where the two side channels are choking it. You see the knot where they crisscross loosening up, and the winds in the center beginning to flow again. You can do this in fact any time you stretch any part of your body, but especially where you have some kind of problem. And because your thoughts are actually tied to your inner winds . . . " I paused for him.

"Like a rider upon a horse . . . ," he filled it in.

"Then it really is true that *picturing* your back loosening up, getting better again, can actually help it happen, as you do your poses. This is one big secret to how yoga really works.

"Now the Master says too that you have to watch the duration of your breath—how long it takes to get a full breath in, and then a full breath out. Which is to say, how fast you're breathing."

"If the whole point is to have a peaceful effect on the inner winds, then I guess you'd want to breathe as slowly as possible," observed the Captain.

"That's true, but to a point," I went on. "It's not really so important how fast or slow you breathe, but rather that your breathing is deep and rhythmic, without any gasping or panting—no broken starts and stops, no ragged edges. At the beginning, when you're still not used to things, then you'd want to breathe a little faster, or else you'd start gasping, which again would put pressure on the choke-points of your major channels.

"As you get looser and stronger—as you practice, steadily—then you can start slowing your breath down, still trying to make sure that both your in-breaths and your out-breaths are deep and regular. Then if you get into a pose that's still difficult for you, and your body needs more fuel, you purposely speed your deep breaths up to feed it. And so in the end, the point is control—that whether you breathe fast or slow, it's a decision to do so, to get maximum benefit for the channels, wherever you happen to be.

"And then lastly here the Master talks about counting: about ways of measuring how long you maintain a pose, for example; or how long you take to inhale, exhale, or hold a breath. The first one we can do obviously just by counting how many breaths we take holding a finished pose, and different poses are best done for different lengths of time, for a different total number of breaths.

"For most poses, it's enough to hold them for five or six breaths. I remember that when I began doing the poses with my own Teacher, this didn't seem like enough to me—it felt like if I held a pose for a lot more breaths, then my leg or whatever would just stretch out an inch or two more that same day. But that's not the way it works; the only way to stretch the body—and free up the channels—is by slow, steady, brief efforts at points all over the body, day after day; because they're all connected. And of course there are certain poses—like where you put your feet straight up in the air over your shoulders—that only really help the channels if you hold them for a longer count.

"There are other things we have to watch and count too: not just how long we hold a pose, but also how long it takes us to breathe in, or breathe out. This is because, for the poses at least, you get the best rhythm by watching to make sure that your out-breath takes the same time as your in-breath: no longer or shorter.

"You can measure this by counting numbers in your mind, but then you might have trouble paying attention to other things, like whether you 'feel' a channel straightening out as you stretch an arm or leg. One easy option is just to connect to your heartbeat—either to the feel of it beating in your chest, or listening to its count in your ears. And then you can watch to see that your in-breath takes so many heartbeats, and your out-breath takes the same number of heartbeats. This really helps prevent the common mistake of not getting all the old, stale air *out* with every breath; because if you keep this mistake up for a whole session, the extra air kept inside begins again to put pressure on the very places in the channels where we are trying to relieve the pressure.

"This habit of staying aware of the count, of making sure that the out-breath takes the same number of heartbeats as the in-breath, also begins to carry over into your everyday life—say, while you are working at your desk, or facing a tense situation; it relaxes you, and helps keep you from choking off your inner channels in the first place."

The Captain let out a big sigh. "I can hardly remember what pose I'm supposed to do next, and now there's something else I have to think about!"

"Practice," I said, sounding like Katrin to myself. "Practice." And then I took him through some really tough poses, just so I could have the pleasure of stopping him when he started to gasp, to remind him about rhythmic breathing. This is all part of a teacher's job—to keep a student's mind as flexible as their joints, and I thought you should know that too, for the next time your own teacher has you puffing.

13

Silent Sitting

Third Week of May

Coming up the path to the main road that next week I ran into a thin, friendly little boy that I recognized as one of the waifs who brought Busuku his trays of food. He was shy and almost walked by, but I saw his eyes on Long-Life and I knew how to make him stop and talk. I held out my little lion and stroked his back, and let the boy pet him too.

He talked a bit; apparently things were getting a little hard for all of the boys with Busuku locked up for so long. And I couldn't help thinking what a waste it was that they could not be learning something useful, something that would help them for the rest of their lives, and not land them in some jail somewhere.

"So, are we done with all that breathing stuff?" started the Captain. "I really was doing all right on that part before we met, you know."

I shot him a look but could see he was just kidding. I'd wager he had spent the whole week trying to keep an even number of in-breaths and out-breaths whenever he'd had to deal with one of the corporal's emergencies.

"Almost done," I replied. "The Master closes this particular part by adding,

Long and fine.

II.50c"

"What's that supposed to mean?" asked the Captain.

"If you think about it, we've talked about the state of the breath: in or out, stopped or moving. And then we've talked about the mechanics of the breath: location, speed, and measurement. Here now the Master is looking at the breath in a deeper way: as a tool to reach deeper and deeper places.

"You see normally, as you go through a series of poses, you are trying to breathe as 'long' as you can—which is to say, keeping the breaths full and hearty on the way in and on the way out, regardless of how fast you're breathing. This is critical for the desired effect on the inner channels; for fixing problems like your back.

"But there are also poses where the goal is to bring the breath down to a very fine, quiet flow—almost as if you were asleep, or listening quietly to a very lovely piece of music. These are the most important poses of all, because these are the poses where you switch over from working on the channels from the outside to working on the channels from the inside."

"From the inside? I don't get it," admitted the Captain.

I tried to think hard of an example from his everyday world. "Let's say you have a long piece of bamboo that you've hollowed out, and use to bring water into your house from a stream outside."

He nodded, and his look was on me with honest interest. He really did have the instincts of a very good student.

"Then one day the water isn't coming through very well—just sort of a small trickle—and you realize the bamboo pipe is clogged up somewhere with some mud or something. Now if you think about it, there are two different ways you can get at the problem . . . " I waited for him.

"Take a stick and knock on the outside of the pipe—sort of like the way you might loosen up an uncooperative prisoner . . . "

I winced, and unconsciously rubbed the scar on my arm.

"Er . . . sorry," he said sincerely. "Or you could go at it from the inside—you could get a long thin reed say and poke it in the pipe and try to break up the blockage. At some point you might want to blow really hard into the pipe and see if that helps too."

"And here it works just the same," I said. "You see, the poses that I've taught you so far work from the outside: we stretch a part of your body to try to cause a parallel straightening of those subtle channels inside. Or we bend at major joints—which happen to grow anyway where blockages in the channels were already present, even in the womb—and try to help loosen these choke-points; all to get the inner winds, the good ones, moving again.

"But you can also go at it from the inside," I continued. "The goal is to free up the good winds—to get them moving again—but always remember too that the winds are carriers, like horses, and that upon them ride your thoughts. They are inextricably tied to one another: move one, and the other has to move.

"Now doing the poses of yoga as we've been doing them so far—almost like a series of physical exercises—is like knocking on the outside of the pipe to loosen up mud that's blocking the free flow of water inside. We're trying to get the horses—the inner winds—loose and moving freely.

And then well-being, both physical and mental well-being, grows and stays with you, because the source is fixed: the choke-points are released.

"But if you think about it, you could also just get the *rider* to move the *horse*, and not vice versa. That is, you could purposely make contact with the kinds of thoughts that would run through the middle channel, and feed them, and make them strong; and then they'd start to flow freely, dragging the inner winds along with them as they go. The grip of the two side channels would start to loosen, as more of the inner energy leaves the negative areas and flows into the middle. And then the middle channel would get fuller and stronger; better able to resist any future choking from the side channels."

"No choking—then all the points where your body hurts, or where it's getting old, would start to change, and get better. And good thoughts—happy thoughts—would start to grow more and more. It's amazing . . . ," he said.

"What's that?" I asked.

"It's amazing to think that there's a real reason why we all feel *happier* when we feel *better*: that there's actually a place where the physical and the mental cross over. It's so obvious, but it's not something you could ever figure out really on your own."

It *was* amazing; and *he* was amazing for seeing it so quickly. I smiled and took him through his usual series of poses rather lightly, so his body and his winds would loosen up, but without his getting tired. Then I sat him down on one side of the blanket we used to cover the floor during the poses. I had him cross his legs loosely—in a way that would be comfortable for him.

"Something you need to know." I said then. "In the old days, doing the poses had only one goal. The Master mentions this goal when he describes how it is that the poses bring you that well-being which stays with you:

> *They do so*
> *Through a balance*
> *Of effort and relaxation;*
> *And through endless forms*
> *Of balanced meditation.*
>
> II.47

And so, you see, the original purpose of the poses was to make you healthy and strong, and straighten out your thought-winds, to the point where you could meditate well, in a whole variety of different ways—always maintaining a balance between the effort it takes to keep your mind from getting sleepy, and the relaxed feeling you need to settle it down and keep it from thinking of too many other things. And the original poses, the earliest ones, were just different ways of sitting for comfort and steadiness as you meditate."

"So are we going to do *meditation?*" the Captain asked cheerfully.

"Not really," I said.

"*Prayer,* then? Or *contemplation?*"

"Not those either," I replied, staring at the floor, trying to think something out.

"To tell you the truth," I said finally, "I don't feel all that comfortable with calling it any of those three things—because people, just normal people everywhere, have such very different ideas about what it is to do meditation, or prayer, or contemplation. And they already have certain feelings about what they think the three are—but, as you will see, what we are going to do together is something fresh; something exciting, and different: a way that we can work on your back pain from the inside, and get your happy thoughts flowing well. It's actually sort of a *plumbing*, really . . . "

The Captain looked dubious. "I don't think the Master would have approved of your calling it *plumbing*," he said.

I frowned, and finally had to nod in agreement. "Well, what we're going to do is just *sit*. We're going to sit together *silently*." I gazed out the window.

"We are going to do *silent sitting*," I said, "and that's all."

14

Learning
How to Sit

Fourth Week of May

The next day on the way to the station I ran into the boy again, and he had a friend with him. Ostensibly they wanted to pet Long-Life, and both he and they enjoyed it immensely. But I could also tell that the boys were lonely, and bored, without their ringleader and adopted daddy, Busuku. By the end of the week all eight boys in Busuku's little gang were waiting on the path to pet and talk. It became a regular thing, and I got to know their names. The first one I'd met on the path was called Kumara Vira—the Young Warrior—and I found out that he'd been the only one brave enough to deliver the little food packages for Long-Life and me, out behind the jail at night.

That week during our class I led the Captain again through his poses—working from the outside, knocking on the pipes—rather lightly. That way he'd still be fresh when we got down to sitting silently together: to working on the pipes from the inside. But first I had to get him sitting right, and for that I decided the military approach might fit him best.

"Now Captain, sitting in silence together so we can start working on your channels from the inside is never going to work unless you learn first to *sit* properly, just as we re-learned how to stand properly. Because first and foremost, above all, your back absolutely must remain straight. Otherwise you're just choking the channels worse at the very same places we're trying to open up again, and the mental plumbing we do won't work that well anyway. So first . . .

"Back . . . *straight!*" He moved up out of his slouch.

"Shoulders . . . *even!*" That little hunch he had from his bad back disappeared.

"Chin . . . *up!*" It came up, but too far. "Not that high! Just the natural place it would be if you were looking straight ahead at something you were really interested in."

"Face . . . *relaxed!*" He tried, but the daily-work crease between his eyebrows didn't change much. "Special attention to those three points . . . ," I began.

"At the lower forehead, between the eyebrows, and . . . and, oh yes." He pushed the corners of his mouth into a gentle smile with his two first fingers.

"Those really are a key to loosening up the choke-points; I mean it," I said sternly. In reply he gave me the salute I guess they'd taught him at military academy.

"Tongue . . . *relaxed*, in its natural position in the mouth, gently touching the spot above your two front teeth just behind them." His whole face started to relax then.

"Eyes?" he said.

"If you keep them open, it will be distracting. But when you shut them for more than a few seconds, your body thinks it's time to go to sleep, from years and years of conditioning. One thing you can do is just lower your eyelids almost all the way, and leave a little crack there. Then keep your eyes pointed down, but be careful not to peek out at anything—just keep your eyes in that unfocused way they have when you're having a really good daydream, with your eyes open but not really seeing anything—you know what I mean?" He nodded, and his eyes flicked away for a moment to the window; to a daydream he often visited, I think.

"Now you want to get relaxed, and you want your breath coming and going through your nose—in the way that the Master called 'fine.' One way to get down into fine breathing is just to take ten quiet breaths first, counting them carefully. If you lose count, start over again: your mind's not quiet enough for you to sit silently yet.

"Later on you can measure the breath to see if it's getting 'fine': listen carefully for any sound at all from the nostrils—on the outside or the inside—and try to quiet them down below audible. It's considered helpful for directing the inner winds into the middle channel if you count each breath from the *exhale* first, rather than from the inhale. So one whole breath would be an out-breath followed by an in-breath: always retaining a feeling of the energy coming *in* at the end, coming to the middle. So try a few now."

I checked his posture while he was watching his ten breaths, still a little bent forward. When he was done I said, "There's a little trick to make sure you're absolutely straight up and down, and straight forward and back as well.

"Put your palm flat on the floor, and push it down, as if you were trying to push the whole floor into the ground underneath this building."

He pushed a bit. "Harder," I said. He pushed a little more. "*Harder!*" I said again, trying to use Grandmother's voice of command.

He pushed his palm down with force this time, straightening out his elbow and getting his shoulder right over his arm. I grabbed them both and said: "See how well all this lines up—each piece over the other, straight as an arrow—if you push down? Now I want you to do the same with your bottom as you sit: push it down, as if you were trying to shove it through the floor."

He did, and suddenly his head popped up another inch or two; his neck rose gracefully out of his shoulders; and most importantly his bad back with its choke-point straightened up away from his hips.

"That's it. That's it exactly. You may need to do a couple of pushes like that as we sit, because the back is a little lazy at first and likes to slump back to where it was, whenever you're not looking."

"What about my legs?" he asked.

"They're all right just like that, for now—crossed loosely. You could even just sit on a bench or a chair, as long as your feet were flat and your back, neck, and head straight. The point for now is to sit in the one most straight and comfortable position you can, so your mind won't be running off worrying about an ache or pain somewhere as we sit."

"And my hands?" he said finally.

"You can put them on your lap, the right on top of the left, palms up, with the thumbs touching very lightly. Or if it's more comfortable you can also just set them on your knees, palms up or down, with the first finger and the thumb touching lightly.

"All this has a helpful effect on your inner winds, and you can refine it more and more as we go. But it's all just physical; more knocking on the pipe from the outside. The last and most important part of sitting is how you position your thoughts themselves, on the inside."

"I know!" he said brightly. "Sit very still and try to think about nothing at all!"

I smiled at him, as Katrin had smiled at me the day I'd said the same thing. There was so much to tell him, and no knowing how much time we had. But we also needed to focus, to concentrate. It is the dilemma every teacher faces.

"There are many ways of focusing your mind as you sit like this," I began. "Almost all of them involve trying to avoid thinking about too many different things. And some of them include certain kinds of special thoughts that are so wonderful that you may not be aware for a while that you're thinking at all. But thinking about nothing is not a goal; in fact, it's a problem. You really want to be careful not to go off into some kind of dreamy feeling, where you're really just sort of relaxing in a lazy way.

"Rather you want to be bright—alert—focused—happy—engaged; as if you were watching a performance by some actors, and the story is so captivating that you can't even hear it when the person next to you says something to you. Do you see the difference? That's not thinking about nothing, it's thinking about *something*, so deeply and joyfully that it perhaps *feels* as though you were hardly thinking about anything; and certainly your mind is not wandering off to any unrelated thoughts either."

He nodded, thoughtfully. And then he said, "Like how you feel when you're reading a good book, or listening to your favorite song. Almost like you forget to breathe; maybe sometimes you even forget to keep your mouth closed, and you catch yourself drooling on yourself, you're so engrossed in the thing. And that's simply not thinking about anything *else*. It's completely different from that dazed feeling you have when you just woke up, or had too much to drink . . . er, not that you'd know about that, of course."

In fact I didn't. But he got the point, and he got it well.

"So we need to choose a thought, a good thought—a thought you can focus upon, that you can enjoy; and one which shoots right down your middle channel and breaks the blockage out of the bamboo from the inside. A thought that the Master describes when he says,

> *It gives the same effect*
> *As releasing, then storing,*
> *The wind of the breath.*
>
> I.34

The point is that there is one method of working from the inside which gives you the same wonderful results as lots of efforts done from the outside. These outside methods are the poses, which you are learning, or things like special ways of breathing; all of them aimed at releasing the inner winds from the places where they are choked, so they can be stored up instead within the middle channel. And this inner method, it's not thinking about nothing; it's thinking about something, on purpose, in a very focused and happy way."

The Captain didn't actually ask what it was; I think he already knew, something before all memory even. He just nodded in a very peaceful way, and I told him softly to practice the ten breaths, and sitting silently, straightly, until we next met together.

15

Free Kindness

First Week of June

If meeting Busuku's boys on the path every day was
a pleasure to look forward to, coming home to the old
woman's house was the opposite. It's not that the work was
difficult; I was used to hard work, and I tried to earn my
keep and more for my mistress, as a point of honor. But so
often when I arrived back at my little shed and loom I'd
find the Sergeant there too, just off duty, most often already
drunk, just sitting around making drunken small talk with
the woman. And too often I found his eyes on me, and it
scared me.

"It is kindness," said the Captain, first thing.

"It is indeed kindness," I agreed, without much surprise.
"And the Master says,

> *Use kindness;*
> *It makes the mind*
> *Bright and clear*
> *As pure water.*
>
> I.33A"

92

"But how to use it, when I am just sitting here silently?" he asked.

"It is simply one of the most sacred and powerful instructions from all ancient times," I said. "It ties together the breath, that closest sister of the inner winds, and quite nearly the most potent thought of all—*kindness*—sending them combined into a direct attack upon the very essence of the choke-points inside that make us sick and unhappy."

"*Quite nearly* the most potent thought?" asked the Captain. I heard what he was saying: Why not start with *the* most potent thought?

"It's coming," I said, like Katrin used to do. "First things first." Then I took him through some of his poses, almost like putting oil on the axle of a cart before you climb aboard to start a trip. After he had rested and warmed his body down, I had him get in position for silent sitting. He did quite well, even down to trying to push his bottom through the floor to get absolutely straight.

I was really very proud of him, my first real student, because he did the one thing that every successful student of anything has to do: he took what I had taught him home and practiced it there on his own, modestly but very steadily, to the best of his personal capacity. I could not have asked for more.

When he was very still, and his breath nice and quiet, I said, "Look inside of your chest now—where your heart is."

"Inside your heart is a tiny red flame, like the flame at the top of a candle. This flame is the power of our selfishness — the habit we have of taking care of ourselves first, and neglecting what others need or want." I waited for a moment until he had it clear.

"Now pretend that you are sitting right in front of the Sergeant, at his home. But he can't see you; you are invisible." I paused again.

"Look into the Sergeant's heart. Right there in the middle is a dark, rotten little pool of blackness. It is his sadness, it is his pain; it is the reason why he drinks, and it is his drinking." Another pause.

"You want to take this pain away from him, forever. It's the compassion we spoke about before; it is the real reason why you are doing yoga. And you decide that you want to take his black pain away so badly that you would even take it into yourself, if it meant you could save him from it." Pause, a longer pause. Compassion, even pretend compassion, is so hard for us.

"And so you begin to take say seven long, slow breaths. The first time you breathe in, that little evil pool of darkness in the center of the Sergeant's heart stirs and moves; it starts to rise up out of his body, like an ugly cloud of blackness. And as you take more breaths it is sucked up out of his chest, up his throat, and then out of his nostrils. And knowing you would take it on yourself to save him from it, you take all his drunken misery in that little cloud of darkness and you keep breathing, in, and in again, drawing it towards your own face. And then hold it there, just outside your own nostrils." I waited, and watched to see that it was time.

"And now something will happen; it will happen a little quickly, and so you have to concentrate well upon this part. In one breath you will suck the blackness in through your own nose; you will take it upon yourself. The blackness will come down your throat, into your chest, and then slowly— very slowly—it will approach the little red flame of your selfishness: the part of you that would never even imagine taking away someone else's pain, if it meant having it yourself instead.

"And the blackness floats slowly towards the edge of the flame, and then suddenly the black makes contact with the red, and there is a burst of beautiful golden light, like a bolt of lightning shining in the purest gold. And in that moment, because you were willing, in that moment, to swallow all the Sergeant's pain into yourself, the crimson fire of your own selfishness is extinguished, forever. It is gone. And in this explosion too the blackness of the Sergeant's pain is destroyed: destroyed for him, destroyed for you, destroyed forever. For this is the power, the power of the grace of selfless compassion for others.

"And you must know this power, and believe in its power. It is very important that you see, and that you know, that the blackness has been destroyed, in that moment, forever—before you even take your next breath. And then you are only sitting here, with me, silently—and inside of you it is only that golden light, filled everywhere with that golden light.

"Now breathe the darkness in, and see it happen."

He did, and then we sat there, in the golden silence, for the longest time. Time enough for the one tear that came slowly down his cheek to dry.

When we came out of it the Captain smiled at me happily, and gratefully. Then in a moment his eyes wandered off towards the work waiting on his desk. Students can be so transparent sometimes.

"That's only the first half," I said firmly, "and we call it 'taking'—taking away someone else's pain, their problems. But now we need to do the second half, which we call 'giving.' Giving and taking: we need to do both."

He nodded, got himself in position, and resolutely pushed his bottom into the floor. I resisted a giggle. Being the teacher was a little too serious sometimes.

"That first part was compassion; taking away someone's pain," I repeated.

"Excuse me," he said then. "But is it really? Could I ever really take away the Sergeant's pain like that?"

"You could; you will. But not the way you think. It's important to understand how you *will* do it. But that comes later; I promise.

"For now we have to go on to giving—to kindness; and you should know that in his *Short Book* the Master introduces both compassion and kindness together, along with other powerful, inner means of freeing the winds.

"If compassion wants to take away pain, then kindness wants to fill the void which is left when pain is gone: kindness wants to give a person whatever they wish for.

"And so now close your eyes again, and imagine again you are at the Sergeant's house. And you want to fill him with happiness, now that his sadness is gone. It could be any kind of happiness, anything you know he might really like; but I have an idea for a happiness you could give him which would be special, because again it would attack our selfishness—which is quite nearly the most powerful negative thought choking the channels within your bad back."

"That *quite nearly* again," mused the Captain.

"Later; soon," I said again.

"So let's pretend this time that when you breathe out, you are sending a person to his door: your breath is a person, and every time you let your breath go again he steps closer to the front door of the Sergeant's house. And this person is . . . " I couldn't recall.

"Who did you say your boss was again?" I asked.

"Oh him . . . well that would be the Superintendent, off in the capital. Tough as nails, especially if I'm late with one of my reports," breathed the Captain, glancing at his desk again.

"Soon," I said.

"So yes—your breath as it flows out is the Superintendent, and then he is at the Sergeant's door, and he knocks. And the Sergeant opens the door—he's all bright and chipper and freshly washed and dressed neat as a pin now, since you took away his drinking.

"And the morning sun beams in upon his smiling face as the Superintendent greets him good day, and with warm hands pushes a letter into his own hands; and the Sergeant opens it, and nearly falls down with joy and surprise, because . . . "

"Because what?" snapped the Captain, sensing already what was in the letter.

"Because it is an official correspondence from the ministry, proclaiming him the new Captain, in charge of this very facility," I said cheerily.

The Captain's face fell. "Then what . . . then what am I supposed to do?" he blustered.

"That's not the point!" I cried. "Or maybe that's *exactly* the point! Don't you see? You are giving him the one thing that would make him most happy, even if—or *especially* if—it's the one thing that makes *you* most happy: the one thing you'd really rather *keep for yourself.*"

The Captain looked a little confused. "I don't get it," he said. "What's that got to do with fixing my back?"

"It has *everything* to do with fixing your back, you . . . " I stopped myself short of the "you *dolt!*" that Katrin might have used, if rarely.

"Think about it, Captain! Your selfishness never got you anywhere! Taking care of yourself doesn't even . . . doesn't even take care of you, at all! It ties up your channels, stops your winds, makes you hurt, makes you unhappy, makes you get older and older, even makes you . . . makes you die, like that, sitting on your selfishness, defending that most valuable worthless thing there is. I'm telling you a secret! I'm giving you the key! You fix it all from the inside, quick, just like that. But you have to give it up, give it up, and *give*, give everything!"

The Captain raised his eyebrows, and his eyes opened wide. "All right! All right! Calm down, young lady. I'm afraid you'll bust a channel."

He was right; I did my ten quiet breaths, and I calmed down, and then we went through the Sergeant's promotion together, sitting silently. And then, just for good measure, we went to the corporal's house and took the black cloud of his lack of drive and energy out of his heart. By then he was so sharp and motivated that the Superintendent—returning from the Sergeant's—ran into him, was immediately impressed, and took him off to the capital as his own protégé: as the next Superintendent, in fact. It was great fun; free and easy medicine for the inner winds.

16

We Misunderstand
Our World

Second Week of June

I've told you already about that law of yoga, and of life—
that when important good things are starting to happen,
then powerful bad things are stirred up too, and they come
and try to stop the good things. Maybe it has something to
do with the channels beginning to open up, I don't know.
Maybe the bad channels fight back, fighting for their very
existence.

And so on the same night that the Captain and I first
attacked our selfishness together, down inside the channels,
the Sergeant came to the door of the shed, as I slept.

Long-Life growled and I woke up instantly. It was quite
late, and a windy night as the summer rains approached.
The moon though was nearly full, and I could make out
the Sergeant's form in a second. His smell, the smell of the
liquor, seemed to fill the room in that very first moment.
And Long-Life was ready to leap but I caught him by the
end of the little rope I always kept tied around his neck, for
the old lady's sake.

"Don't be afraid," the Sergeant laughed lowly. "Nothing to worry about. Just thought we could talk, and . . . " His outline weaved unsteadily in the doorway, and he stepped inside. He had a clay jug in one hand, and his other hand reached out in the dark, groping. It was too late to try to reason with him.

Long-Life and I had been through a lot together. We had a special sign for emergencies. I would yell a word in our language, *bam!*, and then we'd both be up and gone.

"Long-Life! *Bam!*" I cried, and jumped up from the bed. The Sergeant lunged clumsily; I turned sideways, knocked the loom over on him, and ran to the door. Long-Life flashed under the Sergeant's legs, dragging the rope behind him, and then we were out in the moonlight, headed towards open country.

We just ran, and I thought. There was no way we could head back in the direction of the jail and the main road; too many people there, and dawn wasn't that far away. But working over the fields, the other way, was just as bad; I knew from experience that the tracks would be easy to follow come morning.

And then I remembered something my grandmother used to say, about the best place to hide something being right out in the open. And so I stopped at the bridge, close to the old woman's house, and we both crawled under. We would stay here two, even three days, right in the middle of where the search would begin. And when they were all far away following false trails, we'd choose the quietest way on to Varanasi. I had to leave the book, and the notes. I knew Katrin would have agreed. I would write out as much as I could remember later, when we reached the Teacher.

And so we waited, tense at first, and then dozing off at times. I decided after a while that the Sergeant had probably just gone back home, finished off the jug, and fallen asleep. I curled up tight, pressing my little lion's warmth to my chest, as far back under the bridge as we could squeeze.

Something woke me up, a premonition. I looked out to the side, to where the shadow of the bridge ended, and the moonlight began. There was a tiny sliver of silver there in the light; white, curled like a snake. I stared at it for a moment before I realized what it was: the other end of Long-Life's rope.

I started up to pull it in and then a hand came down off the bridge, lightning fast; the rope snapped tight and Long-Life's little body was ripped from my arms, up to the bridge. I scrambled out into the night.

I can hear Long-Life choking and gasping for life, hanging in the air.

"I will kill him," the Sergeant says.

"I know it."

"You will come with me now, back to the jail. Promise it."

"I promise. Let him go."

And he drops Long-Life into the mud there, convulsing, shuddering, flailing in the mud. And I get down in it too, shaking and trying to tear the rope loose from his neck. And he looks up at me with sad helpless eyes and I take him in my arms like a child and we follow off behind the dark Sergeant, back to our jail.

φ

The Sergeant was up early in the morning, went out for about an hour, and returned with the old woman. When the Captain came in the Sergeant went straight to his office with the woman, and then after a while they came back out, and the woman left—without so much as a glance in my direction. Then the Captain had the Sergeant bring me in and asked him to leave, and shut the door.

"I told you; I told you very clearly, never try to escape."

"But I didn't, sir . . . I just ran away, because . . . "

"Ran away? But not to escape?"

"Not like that, Captain. It was the Sergeant; he was drunk, he came to my room while I was asleep . . . "

"Enough!" he exclaimed. "That's not the way I heard it. I have two witnesses who say you tried to escape."

"Witnesses?"

"The old woman saw you run. She went and found the Sergeant, who did good work to catch you before . . . before others did. You should be grateful to him."

"That is not what happened," I said calmly, a special kind of stillness coming on me, as it did sometimes. "They are lying to you."

The Captain fixed his eyes on me sternly, but the truth was in my own. He looked down. "We shall see. But for now I cannot ignore the word of an officer of the Realm, and of a senior resident of this town."

He looked up at the ceiling with a kind of sadness in his eyes, kept them there for a silent moment, and then brought them back down to my face.

"And so . . . ," he faltered, "and so it is my duty, to inform you that you are now found guilty of breaking the laws of the King in regard to escaping from custody, and will now be held in this facility as a convicted prisoner, for an indefinite length of time."

Explanations, objections, expressions of outrage flew through my mind at this idiotic decision in this idiotic little town with its idiot inept officers. And then the stillness came back and silenced them. This was not what it seemed to be. It had a reason; it had a cause. And now was the time to practice yoga—real yoga—the way my Teacher had trained me to do.

"I see," I said steadily. "Prisoner, here, for an indefinite period of time; perhaps a very long time. I understand."

The Captain cocked his head. "You don't seem to be very concerned."

"Concerned, yes," I replied. "Upset, no."

"And why not?"

"Because it won't change what is happening. But something else will. And so there is something else I have to do to change this."

"Change what?"

I looked around quietly, and the words came to me out of the quiet. "I will . . . I will have to change *this*," I said with an unshakable feeling of confidence, waving my arms around me.

The Captain looked around, despite himself. "Change . . . *this?*" he repeated.

"This—the jail. I will change the jail," I said.

"How?" he said, almost entranced. "How . . . change the jail?"

"I will . . . " The words poured through me, unbeckoned. "I will make *inside* the jail *outside* the jail," I said softly.

The Captain leaned back then, with an unsure smile.

"You mean . . . you mean you will do your best to take all this in a positive light. You will try to imagine, perhaps, that you are somewhere else, even as you sit in your cell."

I fixed a cold look on him, laced of steel, like Katrin's.

"That's not what I said at all, Captain. I said that *I will make* the inside of the jail the outside of the jail. Am I not clear? Do you not understand my words?"

"I do . . . understand . . . *what* you say, but not what it means."

"And until you understand," I said harshly, "you will never understand yoga. You will never understand how it really works. And you will carry your bad back and all the disappointments of your life with you to the grave."

He looked at me with a sadness that said he felt how it was true. And I couldn't just leave him there like that. He was my student, no matter what; we shared that sacred bond already. And he was a human, another living being, in pain: and that bond we had shared for time with no beginning.

"It will come," I said, "I will teach you. Goodness knows we will probably have enough time now." I paused and collected myself. We were about to enter the borders of real yoga. And we had to go carefully.

"You need to hear something now, and then I will leave, and you need to think about it for a while."

He nodded, as though this kind of conversation, under these circumstances, were something that happened to him every day.

"The Master says, in his *Short Book*," I glanced towards those lovely pages, at his elbow, "that—

> *We misunderstand our world:*
> *Things that are not themselves*
> *Seem to us as if they were.*
>
> II.5D"

"You make less and less sense," he said, with a touch of impatience. "Perhaps you really are upset . . . perhaps you need to rest, to think. Let me call . . . "

"*Silence!*" I said. Goodness itself was being born, and wrongness sought to stop it. "The jail! Is the jail . . . is this jail *itself*?"

The captain looked wounded, and then he thought for a moment. "Of course it is," he replied. "Everything . . . everything is itself."

"Meaning?" I demanded.

"Meaning that—in the jail's case, I suppose—that the jail is *itself*, and not something *else*; it is a place where you are put when you've done something wrong, and once you're inside the jail you no longer have any freedom: no freedom to go outside of the jail."

"And so, for example," I returned, "the person inside the jail could never be experiencing perfect freedom there, and the people outside the jail could never be experiencing the torment of absolute bondage there. The inside could never become the outside; the outside could never become the inside.

"Because the inside is *itself*," I breathed, leaning over his desk, into his very eyes. "And the outside is *itself!*" leaning into his very being. "Or so . . . or so it seems," I finished quietly.

And then I stood, and looked down at him. "You may call the Sergeant now," I said.

17

The Pen Again

Third Week of June

I didn't waste any time with the Sergeant. Events had drawn us all now into real yoga—into how yoga actually works. And I wasn't about to upset that happy circumstance over something as insignificant as food. I also didn't want to put Busuku or his lovely boys in any more danger on my account.

"Sergeant," I said calmly, touching his arm again. And he jumped again, and glared at me wickedly.

"I will need food—I will need a way to get food."

He nodded, and his eyes gleamed like a wolf's.

"I need you to get me a loom. Any old loom will do. Even that worn-out one at the woman's house."

He opened his mouth to object. I moved quickly. Thank you, Grandmother.

"You see, if I have a loom here—in my cell—I can start to weave some real rugs. I can weave the kind of rugs we make in my country, in Tibet. They are thicker than five of the old woman's rugs; softer to sit on, with a beauty you cannot imagine. One rug will bring you more money in the market than a dozen of hers."

The Sergeant's mouth closed slowly, and he calculated. He was cruel—or perhaps just in some kind of incredible pain, as cruel people always are—but he was not stupid.

"I suppose that could be arranged," he said slowly.

"And I will need yarn; balls of yarn, in lots of colors."

He hesitated. Selling a rug was one thing. Picking out balls of yarn in the marketplace, surrounded by housewives, was another.

"Just send one of the boys, Ravi," called out Busuku from the other side of the wall.

"Shut up, Busuku," snarled the Sergeant, but I saw in his eyes that he'd do exactly that. And soon the boys began bringing me a tray too, although I must say it was always much smaller than my portly neighbor's.

φ

At our next class I sat the Captain down on his blanket and first we did some silent sitting, working on the giving and taking to help his two men. Then we did a straight hour of some very simple work, just bending toes and fingers, ankles and wrists, shoulders and neck. After his rest at the end he looked bright and refreshed, but then he started to frown a bit.

"Was that . . . was that yoga?" he asked.

I laughed. "Closer to yoga than all the exercises you've been doing, for your particular needs at the moment. But I was afraid not to start you with the exercises you'd probably already seen somewhere; I thought you'd think I didn't know anything about yoga, and then I'd never get my book back, and . . . " I let it go there, and we sat through an awkward pause.

"It's really just another part of yoga," I said finally, "like so many things are. And today we must continue with what we were talking about, because if it is at the bottom of how yoga actually works; and if you understand that, then your back will be healed—and then we, you, can go on and heal the others as well."

The Captain surveyed my face thoughtfully, and said, "I'm glad to continue with that. To tell you the truth, when I got home and tried to think about what was wrong with a thing being itself, I couldn't see it the way I could when you were first saying it."

I nodded. This was the way it went with everyone who tried to learn this crucial idea. At least he was working on it himself, at home. That would help a lot. Then I sat still for a moment and tried to think carefully how Katrin would have expressed it; this had been my Teacher's favorite subject.

"Come sit at the desk," I began, and we settled down across from each other. There was a paper lying there, half covered with the beginnings of a report—I wondered for a moment if I were in there somewhere—and off to one side stood a little clay inkpot, and the Captain's pen. It was like the ones back home—just a thin shaft of fresh bamboo sharpened at one end—and I could see a large jar on the floor filled with others. And as Katrin, that beloved being, had done, I picked up the pen, and held it up between us.

"What is this thing?"

"A pen, of course."

"And is the pen . . . itself?"

"Yes, of course it is."

"Itself, by itself?"

"As all things are," he affirmed.

"There, that's it; you did it, just then," I said.

"Did what?" he asked, his eyes looking around him, ever so slightly.

"You turned it around," I said.

"Turned it around?"

"Your mind—your mind turned it around. And the Master says, as he begins his *Short Book about Yoga*—in perhaps the most important of all the important lines of that wonderful book—he says,

> *Yoga is learning to stop*
> *How the mind*
> *Turns things around.*
>
> I.2"

"I don't under . . . "

Moooo! M-M-Mooo-ooo!

I laughed, as I hadn't laughed in months. At least there was some magic still left in the world. I skipped to the window and looked down, about five feet to the ground. There was a huge black cow, with its head craning up to a straggly little mango tree growing against the wall, trying to strip it of its last few green leaves.

"Corporal! *Corporal!* Front and center!" cried the Captain.

The corporal burst through the door, instantly, as if he might have been leaning up against it all along, eavesdropping on our class.

"Sir!" he gasped importantly.

"Corporal, get outside and remove that cow at my window from the facility grounds. I can hardly hear myself think!"

I saw the corporal instinctively rub his leg. I looked out at the cow. Big; black; huge long black ears bent oddly like crow's wings; a mother, with a full udder and babies to feed—and so persistent, very persistent. It occurred to me that she'd probably kicked the corporal *and* pooped on him.

109

"Captain, sir; no," I pleaded. "It's perfect. We need her for a moment or two."

"Need her—need—that nuisance?" whined my perplexed student.

"Need her, yes," I said again.

"Corporal!" he bellowed again.

"*Sir!*" trumpeted back the young man, with a click of his heels.

"Cancel that order! The cow stays where it is!"

"Stays! Yes! Eating the last tree here! Yes . . . *sir!*"

"And corporal!"

"*Sir!*"

"Do an about-face; go out the door; close the door, softly; step over to the bench on the other side; sit down; and do nothing, absolutely nothing, until I call for you. Am I understood?"

"Sir! Sit and do nothing sir! Right away, sir!" And he was gone, and the two of us sighed in relief.

I leaned out the window, and pulled off a few fat leaves, and threw them over the ground to keep Mrs. Cow engaged. Then I returned quickly to the desk, and held up the pen once more.

"Again. This is . . . "

"A pen."

"Itself."

"Itself."

"And *by* itself."

"How else?"

"Observe," I said; for this was exactly what Katrin had said to me.

"Come, come," I urged the Captain, and we stood side by side and leaned out the window together, close together. And I glanced to the side at the dark black curls of his hair, and his capable features, and suddenly realized that he looked very much like my father. And I felt a pang go through my heart. Almost three years now. Three long years since I'd last seen my family.

"*Chuk, chuk,*" I called to My Lady. She looked up with that grizzled face and spread her floppy ears out uncertainly.

"Oh, I'll not hurt you," I crooned. "Just another treat for you."

I held out the Captain's nice new green bamboo pen. The Captain's eyebrows arched and he began to open his mouth, but it was too late. Her huge slobbery tongue was out and up in a second, enveloping the bamboo. And then there was a crunching sound, and a swallow, followed by that inevitable pleading look for more. I threw her down a few more leaves and hurried the Captain back to the desk. I pulled another pen out of his jar on the floor and held it up.

"Again. What is this?"

"A *pen,*" he insisted, beginning to sound a little defensive.

"Itself?"

"*Itself!*"

"By itself?"

"By itself."

"And so it's a pen to the cow as well."

The Captain looked a little confused. He glanced towards the window and licked his lips. And then he said, a little hesitantly, "I don't think you can say it's a pen to the cow. I don't think she sees . . . saw . . . it as a pen, really."

"On the contrary!" I boomed, trying to imitate Katrin's expression at this same juncture; the face and steel eyes so clear I could almost cry. "Isn't it true that she sees . . . saw . . . it as something different, completely different? Isn't it true that she saw it as *something to eat*?"

"Well yes, I suppose so . . . " he stumbled.

"*Suppose?* Say it! Admit it! It wasn't a pen to her at all!"

"Well no, I guess . . . I mean . . . no, quite right . . . you're quite correct," he admitted.

"So *you* see it as a pen, and *she* sees it as something to eat! And who's right? Which one of you is right? Is it a pen, or is it something to eat? Which one is it *really?*" I insisted.

He looked stumped for a moment and then answered, a little more surely, "I don't think you could say that either one of us was *right*, really. It just looks one way to her, and it looks another way to me.

"I guess you could say that what it is depends on who's looking at it," he concluded, and looked to see if I approved. But he wasn't getting off that easily.

"So then it's *not* a pen," I said.

"Well, not to everyone," he replied.

"And so it's not *itself*; the pen is not *itself*," I dragged him on.

"Well, not itself in *that* sense," he agreed.

"Not itself *by* itself; am I right? Not itself by itself so that even the cow would see it as a pen; am I right?"

"Well I suppose . . . I mean, well, yes, you're right," he said, chewing a little on his bottom lip, thinking hard. I pointed down at his desk. Time to come to his rescue.

"What's that paper?" I asked.

"A report," he replied cautiously, "a report to the Superintendent."

"And is the report itself; is it a report made by itself?"

"Well no," he replied. "I made it a report. I take a blank piece of paper and then I write things on it, and as I write it *becomes* a report. No report is a report *by itself*."

I held up the report in one hand, and the pen in the other. "But don't you see?" I breathed with excitement, the same excitement that had filled my Teacher's face on the day Katrin had taken me down this same path. "Don't you see, that the pen is the same as the report?"

"No, no I don't see," he said, sensing the excitement and frustrated that he couldn't share it.

"The pen . . . the pen is like the report, you see. *You* are making it. *You* are writing it. It's just a little green piece of stick, and then *your* eyes come along, *your* mind comes along, and thinks of it as a pen; turns it into a pen; *makes* it a pen." I paused to see if he could pick up the idea and finish it. And by goodness, he did.

"Ah yes! Ah yes! I see! And the cow . . . her mind is *different*, you see . . . and her mind makes the same green stick into *something to eat*. And if it was a pen—if it was a pen itself, *by* itself—well then she'd see it as a pen too, and she'd never even think to eat it.

"*Things are not themselves*," he whispered. "Amazing! I never thought of that!" And then after a long pause he added, "But what's this got to do with fixing my bad back?" he asked.

"Everything," I replied.

"Later," he laughed.

"Think on it," I said, and returned to my cell, where the inside had just begun to become the outside.

18

Out There, Over There

Fourth Week of June

"You remember I said there was one worst thought—worse even than selfishness; the *root* of selfishness really—and that it blocks up the winds in the channels, and causes the pain in your back: causes *every* form of pain, really, physical or mental."

"You did speak of that," said the Captain.

"Well that's it—that's the thought. It's the way of thinking that turns things around; and the Master is saying that the very purpose and meaning of yoga is to stop this way of thinking."

"Well," he observed, "it makes sense that the goal of yoga would be to stop a way of thinking that ties up your channels, and causes problems like my back. That would make the poses—the exercises which we usually think of as yoga—sort of a partner working for the same goal: knocking at the pipes from the outside, while we fix the wind-thoughts on the inside."

"Exactly," I replied, and waited for the question.

"There's one thing that bothers me though," he continued. "I can see how sitting quietly every day and practicing scenes in my mind where I take problems away from others, and then destroy them inside my heart, could have a powerful effect on those inner winds—especially if they are tied to my thoughts. And the same for mentally sending people the things I think they'd most like. But I don't see how the thing with the pen ties in the same way.

"I mean, I realize that there's something about my own mind that makes me see a particular piece of green stick as a pen. And I realize that there's something about that blasted cow's mind that makes her see the same stick as something she might like for dessert.

"And so I realize that the pen wasn't the way I thought it was; I mean, I see that there's a part of my mind that's always been turning things around, in a way: making me think things are themselves by themselves, when really things are themselves only because my mind *draws* them in a certain way.

"But I don't see any clear plan of action, like I did with practicing thoughts of kindness, for example. I don't see anything I could practice and get better at, and which would make *me* get better, the way that say doing the poses every day has helped me."

And when he said that, it suddenly dawned on both of us that he really was getting much better. He hardly ever held his back with his hand any more as he talked. The bags under his eyes were fading away; he was sleeping again. The problem with getting well sometimes is that it doesn't announce itself say the way that *hurting* your back does in the first place. Ah, yoga teachers, even when they succeed with someone, are so rarely appreciated.

"You need to see the larger picture," I answered, "and then we'll have a plan of action—one that actually goes to the core of why your back hurts at all."

"I thought that was the channels," he said. "The channels, and those inner winds, and things getting choked up. I thought that was at the bottom of everything."

"Well, there's bottoms, and there's bottoms." I said. "We just have to keep going until we really get to the bottom.

"So we'll start from the beginning," I said. "Let's start from the womb. Let's start way back at your mother's womb."

He settled back to listen, fixing his eyes on me carefully.

"Now again, that worst of all bad thoughts—the worst of all *ways* of thinking, really—is thinking that things could be themselves by themselves. It is what the Master called 'misunderstanding our world,' and it's the worst kind of thought because it chokes up your channels, and lies at the bottom of every other negative thought that chokes the channels. And ultimately these choke-points are what cause every kind of sickness, and sadness too.

"The first thing you need to know about this habit of misunderstanding everything around us is that we were born with it. Everybody has it, from the womb. In a very subtle way it actually *shapes* our development in the womb, since at that stage it is already causing choke-points, around which important features of our bodies form . . . "

"Like layers of ice forming over the contours of a twig," completed my brilliant student. And I gave him a brilliant smile of encouragement. He really was doing so well, with both the yoga *and* the ideas behind it.

"And even in the womb, even in the very first thoughts we have there—basic impressions of the warmth or pressure inside our mother—this way of thinking begins to assert itself again, and it infects every single thought or perception we will ever have for the rest of our lives.

"At this stage, when it goes from being a seed to being a large, active part of our minds, we give it a special name: you can call it 'selfness.' The Master describes it like this:

> *Selfness is where*
> *The strong impression*
> *Of someone seeing something*
> *And the something someone sees*
> *Makes it seem as if*
> *Each one were itself.*
>
> II.6"

"Whew!" said the Captain. "That's a little much!"

"Looks like that, but not really," I said. "I'll be quiet for a moment; don't be lazy and wait for me to explain everything. I want you to try to tell me what you think it means."

And so we sat for a moment, and he really thought about how his world was really happening to him. Such a precious moment; so rare for us once we grow up into adults.

"I think I've got it," he said finally, trying to hold on to his young ideas.

"Go ahead," I said softly.

"Well it's so *strong*, you see, and I think that's what the Master is saying first of all. I mean, when you first held the pen up, and asked me what it was, I didn't have the vaguest feeling that *my* mind could be playing a constant role in making it a pen. It just looked like it was over *there*," he laid his hand upon the pen on his desk, "and that I was over *here*," he put his other hand to his chest.

"And so each one of us just looked like—well, like *ourselves*, really—the pen being itself out there, being looked at; and me being myself over here, looking at it. I mean that impression, that sense of division is so strong that until you made that big point with the cow I simply never realized that *I* make the pen itself; *my mind* makes the pen a pen, just as the cow's mind draws the same green stick as something good to eat."

"I couldn't have said it better myself!" I cried. "Now think on that for the next week; chew on it."

"Didn't think of it as something to eat," he grinned.

I gave him back one of Katrin's dour old smiles. "Try to catch yourself doing it, from time to time, during the day: turning things around. Your mind is making you see them as they are. But just because they're *out there*," I pointed, "over there," I pointed, "then it makes us think they are what they are *themselves, by themselves,* from *their* side.

"Try it?" I asked.

"Try it," he answered. The Captain was being such a good boy that I treated him to a monster yoga session, until he was standing in a good-sized pool of sweat. And yes, what a teacher sees as a treat may not look like a treat to the student, you see. Have to watch out for that idea of *selfness* about things, we do.

19

Even for Those Who Understand

First Week of July

"I want to check on something," I said to the Captain at our next class. "Something about that idea of selfness."

"Go ahead," he said with confidence. He'd been practicing, I could tell: looking at the things around him; considering how completely different they might look, and therefore *be*, to other people or creatures; and realizing that it was really something in his *own* mind that made them what they were to himself.

"When I say the idea of *selfness* is a mistake that we make all day long, you know I'm talking about everything around us, right? I mean, thinking that a pen is itself by it*self*; that your desk is itself by it*self*; and so on. I don't mean the idea of 'selfness' just about *your*self, right?"

"Yes, of course," he said. "But of course it does apply to *my*self, and to other people too, doesn't it?"

It was a statement, not a question. I let him follow his thought further.

"I mean, I was thinking about it. Like we could take the corporal, for example. Or more specifically, the way the corporal talks.

"Now when I hear him talk, and he talks so slowly and simply, it drives me crazy. I can hardly remember the first half of one of his sentences by the time he's got around to the second half: he really feels like he has to go step by step, very deliberately, until he's said what he has to say. And it annoys me to no end that he can't seem to make a leap or twist of thought.

"But that same way of expressing himself, you see, might strike someone else as very straightforward, and reassuring. I would guess for example that his Mother might see it that way.

"And so can we say that each person's mind is also making them see the people around them—and even themselves—as they are? That people are no more them*selves* than things are themselves *by* themselves?"

"Perfect," I said. "And I'll tell you something very important, although it's not really what we need to cover today. Do you remember back when we talked about the channels of the sun and moon? About the two channels that run down your back, on either side of the main channel?"

"I recall," he said. "They were the bad guys, full of bad thoughts, negative thoughts—and the more full they get, the more choke-points they cause."

"Right; and now you understand something more about them. When you look at *some thing around you* and feel like it has to be itself *by* itself—that it can't be your own mind *making* it look the way it looks to you—then the thought-winds in the sun channel are stirred up, and start to choke your health and happiness. And when you look at people, or at their thoughts themselves, you see—and even at yourself and your own thoughts—and feel like *they* are the way they are by themselves, and not because *your own mind* is seeing them that way, well then it stirs up the winds in your moon channel, and *it* starts to choke you."

The Captain looked for a moment like he'd eaten a very large lunch. But I gave him a minute or two to go over it again; he even swallowed largely once or twice, and then seemed to achieve some kind of idea digestion.

And then the question came.

"But we—but most of us—and if you were right when you said we were born thinking this way—we think this wrong way *all the time*," he breathed.

"We do," I said simply. "And it begins to choke us, even from the womb. Didn't you ever wonder what makes people get older?"

He stared at me, as the implications began to dawn on him. And I left it at that for the moment: as a seed which would blossom into the most beautiful flower of all.

"But let's get back on track," I began. "And I'm glad you brought up that thing about the difference between how the corporal looks to you, and how he looks to his mother.

"And just to check one thing on that: is the way you see him right, or is the way his mother sees him right? Pen . . . or something good to eat?" I asked, pointing to the *green bamboo stick* on his desk.

"Depends on who's looking!" he answered, adroitly.

"Or you could say," he was showing off now, "that the corporal is *neither* way, *by himself*; or *both* ways, to *different* people." I raised an eyebrow in admiration, and took him on further.

"But now you see, when we get to things that we feel strongly about—things that either really hurt us or make us feel good—then that feeling that they are the way they are *by themselves, from their own side*, it gets very strong, you see, and starts to cause real problems. And then what we were calling 'misunderstanding your world' as a seed and 'the idea of selfness' as it began to take hold of your mind even in the womb graduates to a whole different negative way of thinking: to something we call 'grasping.' And the Master explains grasping like this:

> *Grasping is a thought*
> *That comes on all of its own,*
> *Even for those who understand,*
> *And then grows ever stronger.*
>
> II.9

You see, when something really annoys you—like the way the corporal speaks—then it's very difficult to keep in mind this idea that it's your own mind that's making you see it that way, even if you already understand this idea very clearly. If you stop and think about it, if you reflect on it, then you know that the way the corporal talks is actually just like the pen, because . . . " I waited for him to fill it in.

"Because there's the example of the way his mother feels about this very same thing: she loves it. Which proves that the way the corporal talks can't be annoying *or* loveable, from its own side, by itself. My mind makes me see it as annoying; her mind makes her see it as endearing," concluded the Captain.

"Exactly; but we tend to forget all that when something makes us either very happy or very unhappy. And then that old misunderstanding comes up in us almost automatically, all on its own. We feel like the corporal *must* be irritating from his own side, by himself, and not because our mind is making us see it that way: we *grasp* to that feeling.

"And if you think about it, it's a lot easier to get upset if someone *steps* on your toe, than if you stub it yourself. If you can keep in mind that it's your own mind making you see the corporal as annoying, you might be able to stop yourself from getting upset . . . "

"Choking your channels, hurting yourself . . . ," he added.

"Right. But even people who understand all this, they forget, and then their feelings start to escalate, start to get stronger, and then . . . ," I paused.

"Later?" he asked.

"Later," I nodded. "Cook that for a week, and then we'll go on." And then we did our giving and taking, and our poses, regular as clockwork.

20

Fist and Lightning

Second Week of July

I knew that this next class would be important; I knew it would take us to another level entirely. And so after some silent sitting on giving and taking, I had the Captain go through his poses first, and for the most part I was silent, just counting out his breaths for him at a medium pace. I knew he would take this as a treat and that he'd feel fresh when our talk continued, about how yoga really works.

"And so you see, our inborn tendency to misunderstand the people and things around us escalates to a new level, when something seems either very pleasant or very unpleasant to us. We lose control of ourselves, even if we already have some understanding, and the last thing in the world we can do at that moment of emotion is to recall that it is actually *our own minds* making us see this thing the way we do. We are stubbing our own toe, but we feel strongly that someone else must be stepping on it: we grasp to that mistaken notion. And then this triggers, very quickly, a very wrong chain of events. As the Master puts it,

124

Assailed by what feels good,
We begin to like things.
Assailed by what feels bad,
We begin to dislike things.

II.7,8

If you really believe that someone has stepped on your toe—if you grasp to the notion that the corporal is irritating *in and of himself,* and not because *your own mind is making you see him that way*—then in the very next moment you begin to feel strong feelings of dislike for this other person. And it works the other way too: the moment you grasp to the idea that another person is nice from their own side—by themselves, and not because *your* mind is making you see them that way—then you start to have a strong feeling of liking them."

"So is it wrong to *like* things?" interjected the Captain.

"I didn't say that; I didn't say that at all," I objected. "Nor would the Master ever say that. We *do* like things; we *should* like things. All of us enjoy beauty: the beauty of a sunset; the beauty of a flower; the beauty of a young child's smile . . . " And here the Captain's face fell, strangely.

"Who could say it would be wrong to like it if the Sergeant were cured of his drinking, and the corporal were freed from his lack of energy? And who could say on the other hand that it's wrong to *dislike* the pain you feel in your back—or the pain being felt in the entire world at this moment, for that matter—and want to end them both, forever? Why, it is the very purpose of yoga, and you know that: it is why we are here, and your heart tells you so.

"No, it is not the emotions of liking and disliking that are wrong themselves; rather, it is a *certain kind* of liking, and a

125

certain kind of disliking. It is liking something *the wrong way;* it is disliking something *the wrong way*. It is *misunderstanding* pleasure or pain; it is a feeling that pleasure or pain happen by *themselves,* from their own side; it is grasping to them desperately this way, forgetting that they appear to you as they do only because *your* mind *makes you see them* as a pleasure or pain."

There was a long pause. "But I don't really see the difference," said the Captain. "Pleasure or pain—whether it exists out there by itself, from its own side, or whether it's something that my own mind is making me see—still we like the pleasure, and dislike the pain, just the same."

"Not the same," I hissed, and it felt as if Katrin had taken over my mouth; my mind; my very being.

"If you stub your own toe," I said, "do you stand and strike your own face with your fist?"

The Captain stared at me, in a trance. It all began to dawn on him.

φ

Power attracts power. When one tree grows tall above the others, lightning comes to strike it. And so as the Captain and I were on the verge of understanding how yoga really works, things fell apart.

The Sergeant went out in the late evening, and didn't return for hours. When he did I was sleeping, but I heard him come in. He didn't go to the room on the side to sleep; instead he sat down on the bench there against the wall. The moon was out, and a pale light was coming in through my window, surrounding me. And although he was in the dark beyond the moonlight I could hear him, drinking slowly from a jug, and setting it back on the bench, and then drinking again. And I felt his eyes upon me as he drank.

And then there was a shuffle, and he got to his feet. A thrill of fear went through me. He walked up close to the bars, and I could see his tortured face, and the red glow of his eyes, and the shadows of the bars throwing dark black lines across his body. And then his hand was on the crossbar, and he slid it open, and came to me.

I scrambled up and crouched there, on the floor.

"Nowhere to run, this time," he breathed. He started towards me, and I backed into the darkness of the corner, still crouched like a cat.

He stood there in the moonlight and tapped his stick on the floor.

"Out here, girl," he said, his tone growing ugly. "You know what this feels like." He struck the stick once more to the ground, with a loud crack.

I shook my head; I saw the very ends of my long black hair brush through the edge of the moonlight, and then before they settled back on me the end of his stick flew out, thrust straight into my belly. I cried out in pain.

"Out here! Now!" he roared.

I was shaking all over. I could hardly think. But I knew I would not move an inch to him while I still breathed.

The stick made that sickening *whoosh* through the air and caught me across the face. The blood wet my lips; I licked it dumbly. Long-Life began to bark furiously, on the other side of the wall.

"Now! Now!" he was screaming. And the stick flew again, and it came to me in a haze that I had to cover up, like Busuku had said to do. And more blows came but I turned and crawled into the corner and then he tore at my hair with his hands and a chunk ripped out but I curled up tighter with my hands around my hair and my dress and then Busuku is screaming "Ravi! Ravi! What are you doing!" And then the stick is just coming down *whoosh, whoosh,* one

127

after another on my back and the Sergeant is raging with curses and Long-Life is howling my pain for me and Busuku is tearing at the bars of his cell and crying "No! No! No!," but I just go quietly into my mind, to where the Master's *Short Book* lies, and I begin to sing the verses softly to myself, to the rhythm of the blows.

And I was somewhere in the second chapter, I remember, when he stopped from sheer exhaustion. And he dropped his stick and stumbled back to his room there, and fell asleep.

21

Truly, Everything Is Suffering

Third Week of July

When the Captain came in with the morning light, the corporal took him silently by the arm and brought him to the door of my cell, still thrown open. And I was still curled up, but I had fallen out of the corner onto the floor, near the stick.

I opened my eyes. I could see the Captain's feet. And there was a voice, Busuku's voice, but it sounded like the voice of a King, and not a criminal.

"Captain," he said evenly. "If you possess . . . within you . . . still . . . any single shred . . . of integrity . . . then you will . . . *discipline* . . . your man. Now."

I heard the Captain's breath catch in his throat. I saw a hand come down, near my face, and close around the stick. The knuckles were white, pure white.

And then I could hear the Captain dragging the Sergeant out of the side room with silent rage, and the Sergeant protesting weakly, half asleep still, and then he was thrown on the floor beside me, gasping for breath, and I could see his face down there close to mine, full of fear, trembling.

"Sergeant, stand up." He just closed his eyes, and shook his head. I still couldn't move. All I could see of the Captain was his feet, and the end of the stick, that evil thing, against the floor.

"Stand up and remove your shirt. That's an order. *Now!*" screamed the Captain.

The Sergeant didn't even open his eyes. The Captain's hand came down on his collar and ripped the shirt off his back in a single burst of rage.

I saw the end of the stick come up off the ground. I said, to the floor, "*No.*" And I tried to turn my head up, and I did. And I saw the Captain's terrible face, and the stick—poised, in the air.

"*No,*" I repeated, looking him in the eye. And his anger turned to me.

"*Silence!*"

"No, I will *not* be silent," I whispered. "I am your teacher, and I say: No. Put the stick down."

The blood drained the rage in his face to a pure fury. "*I* am in charge here! *I* am the Captain!"

"No," I said again. "Remember your yoga. Remember what makes you see him like this."

"I have seen! I see! I can see!" he roared again, and the stick came up and I threw my body forward over the Sergeant's. I covered him, like my child, and I felt the warmth there amidst the trembling and the stink of liquor.

"Get up! Get off of him!" It didn't even sound like the Captain now. The voice was high, hysterical, like a little boy lost in a tantrum.

"Remember your yoga," I cried out once again.

"Remember this!" And the stick came down hard, against the floor, within an inch of my head. And I could hear the Captain, sobbing now, and he sucked his breath in once, just once, and he screamed with all his might *Damn!* and the stick came down on my back once; *Your!* a second time; *Yoga!* a third time.

And my eyes were shut dark in the pain but I heard him throw the stick down and run outside towards the road sobbing in pain and there was the precious little warmth below me, safe, and the warmth of the new blood coming down my back, and I took my rest within the warmth.

And after a while in the silence the Sergeant stirred, and he crawled out from beneath me, to the door, and out the cell. And he stayed there on his knees and turned around and stared at me, grasping the bars with his forehead up against them, as if he were on the inside, and I were on the outside.

I closed my eyes and went back to the Master's book, to the place I'd left off the night before. And it said,

> *Truly,*
> *Every part of our lives*
> *Is suffering.*
>
> II.15c

22

A Vessel

Fourth Week of July

That first day I simply laid on the floor of my cell, on my stomach. I was terribly thirsty. At some point the corporal came in, held up my head, and helped me drink some water. He looked like he'd been crying, and he was alone.

I slept until late in the evening, and then I heard footsteps, or rather felt them, with my cheek on the floor. And someone spoke, and it was the Sergeant, but I was too far gone to be frightened.

"Girl, oh . . . girl . . . don't be afraid now."

I tried to look up, but I couldn't. I saw his hands come down, and they set a small clay jar on the floor, and next to it a little dish of something.

"Hold still now; we have to move these things." I felt him take my hair gently in his two hands, and pull it up off my back, out off the drying mass of blood and pus. And then I felt him carefully separating the pieces of my dress in the back, pulling them down to my waist.

"Now this part will hurt, so get yourself ready," he said. "But it has to be done.

"I know . . . ," he said then, faltering. "I know . . . how this has to be done . . . to heal. I have . . . seen it . . . before, once . . . " And he poured strong liquor from the jug across my back, and it hurt like fire, but I was too tired to cry out.

And then he took the little dish in his hands and slowly daubed something into the cuts across my back; it felt cool, like ice from the mountains of my homeland, and it smelled like sandalwood, and fresh butter.

And when he was done he set a clean white cloth across my back, softly. He stood, and picked up the jug, and there was a pause. And then I heard him empty the rest of the liquor out into the other filth at the hole in the back wall.

And then he was gone, and I slept soundly, and the wounds began their healing.

φ

It was only after three days that the Captain returned; he came straight to my door—I was sitting up on the floor—and asked me if I felt strong enough to come talk at least in his room. And I did, and I came.

He sat at his desk and I sat down stiffly across from him; he pretended not to notice and said, "Well now, I was giving some more thought to those ideas, and . . . " He stopped at the look in my face.

"Captain, we can't just forget everything and go on like that."

His face reddened, and his eyes dropped to the floor. "I know," he said finally. "I am really very sorry . . . very sorry for . . . for having hit you."

I waited for his eyes to come back up to mine, and there was a pause—some tension. And then I gazed out the window.

"It's not really that you hit me," I said finally, trying to sort the thoughts out myself. "That's not what's wrong." And I thought again for a moment.

"You see, it's not that you made a mistake. Every student makes mistakes with their teacher; it's part of being a student. If the student never made any mistakes, then— you see—they wouldn't really need a teacher in the first place. And so mistakes, mistakes like what you did, they are normal, and a real teacher doesn't let them get in the way. No; it's something else," and I frowned a bit, and then it came clear to me.

"The problem is, you see, well, it's something the Master says himself, in the *Short Book*. He says,

> *And another way*
> *Is to ask the Master*
> *For their blessing.*
>
> ɪ.23"

"Another way . . . for what?" asked the Captain.

"Another way for reaching the highest goals of yoga: just before this verse, Master Patanjali has listed some powerful methods of reaching pure happiness, and perfect physical health. And then out of the blue he says, 'But you could do the same thing, just by asking the Master for their blessing.'"

"But I thought *he* was the Master; is there some *other* Master here?"

"He is talking about the Master that every student has: he is talking about your own teacher."

I had reached the Captain's pride again, and it was no small amount of pride—I suppose it's the same really with any talented pupil, and it's the teacher's job to pull it out, beat it with their own kind of stick, and then put it back in the student's heart as a healthy kind of confidence. And so we began the process.

His eyebrows arched up. "I'm not sure," he began, "I'm not sure I could call you . . . a *master,*" he said. "Why, you're not much more than a girl, really."

I reached in and cooled my own rising emotions. And then I nodded, slowly. "No, no, I really am not a master."

He nodded back, as if the point were finished.

"But I am . . . I *am* your teacher," I added.

His eyes narrowed; he was getting upset. I would have to do this carefully.

"You are *teaching* me, a little; yes, that's true," he said flatly. "But it's only because I have asked you to; it's only because *I* have arranged for these . . . these sessions, shall we say."

I smiled, but it hurt a bit. He didn't even want to call them classes. I said, "And so really . . . what you're really trying to say, is that *you* are the Master here; that *you* are the Master of these . . . classes . . . because it is you who has decided to have them. And then I, I am just someone, someone that you use to give you the classes: you employ me in that capacity, and so in a sense I am . . . shall we say, your *employee,* and not your teacher."

His eyes fixed on me, smoldering. The silence said that, well, essentially, that was exactly the way it was.

"And that's the problem, you see," I said gently, straining to be heard. "Yoga . . . yoga cannot be taught that way. Even if this place were some fancy school; even if I owned it, and you came here for classes; even if you were *paying* me in some way, still the yoga would never come to you—I could never *grant* you the yoga, you see, even if I wanted to and tried to—unless you regarded me as a teacher should be regarded. And that is with respect, with deep respect.

"Oh it's not that teachers are some kind of faultless beings; it's not that we're not susceptible to our own problems, or that students should follow their teachers blindly.

"But we are, you see, *vessels*; we hold something inside us which is bigger and much more beautiful than us as individuals. Yoga, you see, it began back—long back, long long before even the Master first wrote it down. And it has been passed down—poured from vessel to vessel, poured from teacher to student, and then to their students—for hundreds and hundreds of centuries. It has survived not just in books but in living persons, in the words and touch and thoughts shared between living beings: something beyond what a book can ever do.

"And if books are precious, and they are—precious beyond all measure, the combined knowledge of generation after generation of effort and pain, mistake and discovery— then our teachers are so much more. For regardless of what we think of a teacher, regardless of the weaknesses and faults we may see in them, they are still the one and only door we have to the living experience of countless generations of teachers who came before. Ultimately every teacher contains the knowledge of all the teachers before them; ultimately even someone as young and inexperienced as me holds the very water that was poured into Master Patanjali by his own Master, and which he poured into his own students. And in that sense, yes, I am a master too; I am *your* Master, because I am your teacher."

He started to say something, but I held up my hand. "Again, I want you to know. I don't mean 'Master' in a religious sense, say. I don't mean that you should bow to me or give me things or anything like that. What I *do* mean is that you should *respect* me, *respect* me, not for me, but for yourself. It is the kind of respect and affection that one would have for a doctor who has been your doctor for your whole life; who has seen you through everything from baby colds to the more serious illnesses that strike us over our lifetimes.

"And when a patient or a student has this kind of regard or respect for the doctor or the teacher—and I mean no matter *what* the teacher is teaching them—then something happens: a magic, a kind of magic is let loose. A 'blessing,' the Master calls it. All the power of the healing, all the power of generation upon generation of people who struggled to learn and then learned and then granted that great gift onto the next generation, so it would live—so *they* could live—all that power is released to you.

"And then, you see, the healing will happen. The yoga will work. And otherwise—if you . . . if you *think* of me the way you have been doing, and I'm not talking about mistakes that happen like that with the stick, in my cell—but if you don't *respect* me, as a teacher, as *your* teacher, then you will never get better. And one day you will just lose interest, and go on to something else, and never find out how much farther this healing can go. Not to mention . . . " I paused to see if he would pick it up.

"Not to mention my two men," he said softly. "Whose pain has become . . . even more difficult . . . to ignore." He sighed and looked down at the ground. The sweetness of the truth went to his pride, and they began their struggle. I cheered our side on silently, and it was a long few minutes, and then his eyes cleared and I knew we had won.

"Corporal!" he called to the door.

The door fell open, and the corporal fell in behind it. He picked himself up clumsily and dusted off his trousers.

"Sir! Ah . . . sorry, sir!"

"No problem, corporal. Tell me, is the Sergeant still here?"

"He is, sir! Right . . . er . . . right outside the door, in fact . . . sir!"

The Captain rolled his eyes a bit at the privacy no one in a jail ever knows. "Ask him to come in," he said.

They came, and stood at the side of the desk. The Sergeant was completely sober but pale from the effort I think, and his hands were shaking slightly. He glanced once over at the Captain's stick, leaning in the corner.

"Men," began the Captain, "I . . . I have something to say. And I . . . I wanted to say it in front of you too. I . . . I wanted you to hear it too."

The pair stood there, still as stones, and nodded dumbly. I had a strong feeling that this was the first time in all these years that the three of them had ever spoken together, as a group.

"Now . . . what I wanted to say was . . . was," he sighed, and gulped down a breath, looked up once to the ceiling or somewhere past that, and then said quickly, "I wanted to say, in front of you both, that I . . . that I am very sorry for . . . for what happened the other day, when I . . . when I lost my temper, and took the Sergeant's stick and hit . . . "

He paused. It was hard for him, very hard I knew.

"And hit . . . " he said resolutely, "my . . . my . . . *teacher*," the word came out once, and then it was easier.

"My teacher, Miss . . . Miss . . . "

He stopped abruptly, and I feared for the worst. I glanced at the Sergeant and the corporal. They were glancing nervously at me. And then we all looked back at the Captain.

"Why," he blurted out, "why, I don't . . . *I don't even know your name!*"

I was stunned for a moment. "Well, why . . . why, it's Friday," I said.

"No, no," he said back to me. "Your name . . . I need to know your name. I already know what day it is."

"Oh no," I stumbled. "I mean, you see, my name—it's my name, you see; my name—it's—Friday."

The Captain sat with his mouth open for a moment, and finally it sunk in. "Oh! Oh! I see! Well then, well then, men, I want you to know, that I . . . that I'm, well, apologizing. I'm apologizing to . . . Miss Friday; to my *teacher*, Miss Friday."

The Sergeant and the corporal stood dumbstruck, their mouths still open. And then the Captain came back to himself and thundered, "Sergeant! Corporal! Have you no work to do? Duty . . . er . . . duty, calls! Dismissed!"

And they fell out the door almost the same way they'd fallen in; and we did our giving and taking for them; and then last I took my new student through a series of poses designed to make him nearly as sore as I was.

23

Pride Before a Fall

First Week of August

A week later I was just walking into the Captain's room for class when the corporal burst in past me, brushing against my back. I winced; the yoga I did every day had probably kept me from being crippled, but things still took time.

"*Pig!*" cried the corporal.

"*What?*" roared the Captain.

"I mean . . . Pig! *Sir!*" returned the corporal.

"*What?*" the Captain again.

"Pig! Big pig! *Sir!*"

"Corporal, *what . . . pig!*"

"Big pig, sir! Big pig on the front porch! Can't get him off, sir!"

"For goodness' sake, corporal. If you can't get a pig . . . "

"*Big* pig, sir!"

"If you can't get . . . get a *big* pig off the porch, corporal, then for goodness' sake, just ask the Sergeant to come out and take care of it, like . . . like he always does," he said, throwing a glance in my direction.

The corporal stood silent for a moment, his mouth working, but nothing coming out.

"Ah . . . sir, the Sergeant, sir, the Sergeant is already on the scene . . . on the scene of the incident, sir!"

"Then . . . then just tell him to . . . you know, to . . . ah . . . to do his thing, you know," the Captain looked over at me significantly, but as usual it went over the corporal's head directly.

"Not possible, sir! You see sir, the Sergeant . . . the Sergeant, sir, I believe he has . . . he has *burned his stick*, sir! Sir!" And with that the corporal peered out the door, to see if the Sergeant might have heard. I imagined that even without a stick the Sergeant knew how to express his dissatisfaction over someone snitching on him to the Captain.

"Oh blast it!" exclaimed the Captain, and he sailed out to the porch with the corporal and I in his wake; asked the Sergeant to step aside; and leaned down and threw his arms around what really was a rather immense pig.

"Sir!" cried the corporal.

"Your back!" cried the Sergeant.

And the Captain just squatted down in a nice Uneven Pose and hefted up the beast and carried him out to the road and sent him on his way. He walked to the porch with a huge smile, stopped there near the bottom of the steps to slap some non-existent dust off his hands as his two admirers looked on, and then for good measure threw his foot up high on the railing and fussed with his shoelaces for a moment.

"Back to class!" he grinned at me importantly, and we walked back between the two awestruck assistants to the Captain's room.

Before he had even sat down, I said, "Captain, sir, you shouldn't have done that. You shouldn't have done that at all."

He gave me a surprised look. "Oh, but it was nothing; no problem at all. My back really is doing magnificently, you see."

"I'm not talking about your back," I replied. "I'm talking about your foot. About showing off, when you swung it up so high on the rail, just to show off."

"It wasn't exactly *showing off* . . . ," he began.

"It *was* showing off," I answered, and then I held my hand up to my chin for a moment, thinking how to say it.

"Here, come out here in the middle for a moment," I said, and he came around to stand where he usually did his poses.

"There's something I want you to see. It's a thing called *focus,*" I said. "Now we'll start with the Warrior of Excellence pose: the version where you are standing with your feet wide apart, bending at your knees, and holding your arms out straight to both sides."

He took the pose, and then I said, "Notice first how you feel." But I knew exactly how he felt: straining with his legs and breath, his eyes darting over to me once and then again, to see if it was time to stop yet.

"Hold your head up very straight now, neck as straight as you can make it too, and gaze out towards your hand, steadily." He did so for a whole breath.

"Now focus your gaze on your finger," and another breath passed.

"Then on the tips of your fingers," and I let two breaths pass.

"And now on your fingernails," one more breath. "And then the fingernail of your middle finger only," two more breaths. "And now on the end of that fingernail; on the curve of fingernail at the end." And he did, for three breaths.

"Good," I said, "now relax."

He stood up straight and looked at me steadily. "That's the longest you've ever held that pose," I said. "Twice as long as before, in fact."

He raised his eyebrows. " Sure didn't feel like that," he mused.

"It's the power of focus," I said. "As the Master says,

> *Locking the mind*
> *On an object*
> *Is focus.*
>
> III.1

And once you've chosen the object, and locked in on it, then you try to stay there, stay with it. Then the focus changes into fixation, which the Master describes in the very next line of his book:

> *And staying on that object*
> *Over a stretch of time*
> *Is fixation.*
>
> III.2

Again, you should understand the principle. Remember that the place where body and mind meet is deep within the channels, where your thoughts are riding like horsemen on the inner winds.

"Now normally our thoughts are flying around every which way, flitting from one object to another, like a fly. Land here; touch the object for a second; take off; land on another object, moment by moment, throughout the whole day.

"And this restless flitter of the thoughts is reflected in the inner winds, which then tend to crowd up around the choke-points—tightening the knots there, and ultimately damaging the parts of the body located around each particular choke-point.

"This is precisely why people whose everyday work demands constant bursts of thought in different directions, with constant interruption of their focus, begin over time to exhibit the same sorts of physical problems: problems with their heart; ulcers; even, say, baldness; all connected to certain subtle choke-points that are aggravated by the very disruptions of focus which their work requires.

"It's also why *not* being interrupted for a good period of time—getting a chance to sit down and focus on one thing like a good book or your favorite music for some time—is so relaxing. The focus, and the fixation in the focus—staying there—has a calming effect on the inner winds . . . " I paused.

"Which takes pressure off the choke-points, relaxing their grip on the middle channel; and then happy thoughts are free to flow there again," he finished for me.

"That's the idea," I said. "So you see, focusing the mind, and fixing it there, so it is still, has the same effect on the channels that we are trying to achieve with the yoga, with the poses, in the first place. So if you can do both at the same time—knock on the pipes from the outside, with the poses and a very steady breath—while you work on the inside of the pipes by stilling your mind, by focusing it on one object as you go through the poses, well then it's much, much more powerful. It will make you and your back even more healthy, and calm your mind down too.

"And that's all the trick there is to it: pick a spot to focus on while you hold the pose. Traditionally it could be a part of your body that you're facing anyway—say the tip of your finger, or a toe—but you can also gaze beyond your hand for example to a point on the wall. And then it really is a tremendous help if you narrow down the focus to a *particular* little spot, say part of your fingernail, or a tiny mark on the wall.

"Try very hard to hold your eyes there without moving them the slightest bit during the whole time you hold the pose. This is a very simple and profound way of staking the thoughts down too to a single place; and then later—when you are doing the silent sitting, for example, or even just trying to concentrate on solving a problem at work—you will find that the *habit* of focusing and fixing your mind during the poses carries over to every part of your day, with wonderful results. Because people who can really focus are just better at whatever they do: they succeed more, and they have more fun doing it."

The Captain nodded, and then his forehead creased slightly.

"And oh," I said. "Just to remind you that *while* you focus, you remember to keep those three points very loose: it defeats the purpose if you center in on a point of focus with a frown and a scowl that locks up that very important final intersection of the channels—between your eyebrows, at the lower part of your forehead."

He tried to un-crease his forehead, but the effort to concentrate on this just made the crease deeper. It takes practice.

"You were wondering, I think, what all this has to do with . . . with the pig, I think," I said.

"*Big* pig!" he corrected me, but nodded.

"Well, you see, it's that focusing and fixing the mind is a double-edged sword. If you focus it on something neutral, like a spot on the wall, then it has a very calming effect on your thought-winds.

"And if you go further and focus it say within a choke-point itself, or even better on a kind thought—say on how what you are doing could help the Sergeant, or the corporal—well then even during the poses it has an even more profound effect.

"And ultimately, the Master goes on to say, you could even do these and at the same time go one step further, and focus say on the ideas we were talking about with the pen—on stopping the ultimate negative thoughts that stream constantly through the channels, the side channels. All even as you do the poses. This though takes a little more explaining, and it will come . . . "

"Later," he smiled.

"That's right," I nodded. "But now suppose that instead of focusing on one of these positive things, you focus say on your own leg, and how high you are able to lift it, and how impressed the people who are watching you lift it will be."

The Captain blushed a bit and looked at the floor.

"Well then, ironically, you are sending a negative thought—a thought of pride, a competitive thought— right down to your leg, *just by focusing* on your leg as you entertain the negative thought. Do you see?" I exclaimed. He nodded.

"And then, with your own mind, with your own thoughts of vanity, you are actually starting to damage yourself physically—you are beginning to injure the very part of you that you are vain about.

"And then one day all the negative thoughts and the power of the winds tied to them reaches a level where the very same part of you that you were so vain about gets a new choke-point, and that triggers and actual injury; whether it's a pulled muscle, or a joint popped out of place, or even just some ugly wrinkles say on your face.

"And so it's really true, what they say, about pride coming before a fall. It's not just that the feelings of vanity about how you're getting more slender or more muscular by doing the yoga poses are something unattractive—they are. And it's not just that they distract you from the original goal you have promised yourself to: healing yourself with yoga, so you can help others heal themselves too. It's that doing your yoga *for the wrong reasons*—for self-centered, selfish reasons—can actually *hurt* you, and defeat the very purpose of yoga.

"So; no more showing off?" I concluded.

"I'll . . . try," he smiled, and we did giving and taking for the men, and then some very good yoga together.

24

Next to Godliness

Second Week of August

A few days later, when the Sergeant had gone off to the side room to sleep and all was dark and quiet, something woke me up. It was a noise—the noise of a small creature in pain; it pulled at my heart, and I strained my ears to catch exactly where it was coming from. It sounded as if it were perhaps in Busuku's cell.

I decided to take a chance; if something were really wrong, it was worth the risk of some trouble to find out.

"Busuku . . . Busuku; are you awake?" I whispered.

The little whining noises stopped, and all I could hear then was Busuku's labored breathing.

"Busuku . . . Busuku; are you all right?"

I heard him shift around on the floor, but still no answer. I thought back to lunchtime; Busuku's boys seemed to be doing the cooking themselves, and sometimes they got a little free with the oil and chili peppers. But I didn't recall it being one of those days.

"Busuku . . . ," I whispered once more, a little louder. "What's wrong? Is there anything I can do for you?"

"All right, all right," he said, in a perfectly normal voice. "There is something you can do for me, Miss Friday . . . ," and then there was a mysterious pause. Thoughts flashed through my mind about what my mission might be. Digging through the wall between us to save him from some mortal injury? Breaking out the back window, to fetch help for him from town?

"I need . . . ," he said with a tinge of embarrassment, "I need you to tell me how to do that blasted Western Stretch Pose, you see. I sit down like you said to, and I stick out my legs, but I can hardly touch my knees, much less my toes. Is there some kind of trick to it? Come on, you can tell me. I promise I won't leak it out to anyone else unless I ask you first."

I giggled despite myself. "Busuku, dear Busuku—what are you talking about? How do you know what I said about the Back Stretch Pose? Do the walls of this place have ears?"

"That they do," and I heard a smile in his voice. "I'm surprised you haven't discovered it yet. Now let's see . . . middle cell . . . Miss Friday, go press your ear to the wall about two feet up off the ground, say six inches from the corner where the poop hole is, towards the front."

I did just that, and my jaw dropped. I could distinctly hear snoring—from the Sergeant's room, I guessed—as clear as if I were standing there myself.

"Oh, Busuku! That's wonderful! I can hear the Sergeant, clear as day!"

"Odd thing, too, if you ask me," muttered Busuku. "He's been sleeping like a baby for weeks now. You'd think he was plumb out of money for liquor, but then he's got your rugs to sell, and they bring good money, I tell you. I haven't eaten this well in years."

I smiled to myself again. "Ah now that, Mr. Busuku, may be causing your feet to grow further away from your knees, you see," and I went on to give him a few tips about what he could do to help. Thus began our secret nighttime lessons together; and I was more careful with what I said to the Captain in my other classes, knowing that our audience might be larger than I'd thought.

After we'd finished giving, taking, and the poses that week I sat with the Captain, as usual, to talk a bit. I'd thought of something I'd forgotten to say the week before.

"Captain, there was something more I wanted to mention about the idea of focus," I began.

"I wanted to make sure that you understood, clearly, that focusing in a negative way—in a vain way—on your body as you get stronger and leaner would actually set you back in your progress . . . "

He nodded, "I understand. And you were right. It makes sense. It's one of those things you know by instinct is right, the moment you hear it."

"Good; thank you," I replied. "But I also wanted to say that it's not vain at all to feel an honest happiness—a healthy sort of pride—about the progress you have made, and how good you really do look and feel when you're doing your yoga regularly, and for good reasons: with the idea that you might help others. And then even when others see you, and admire your progress, it's a good thing; you are fulfilling your goal of being an inspiration for them to heal themselves too."

He nodded again, and I have to say that even his face was changing, dramatically. His eyes had a crisp clarity about them, and his skin was fairly gleaming.

"And I was thinking, you know, about the difference," I continued. "Because it's such a fine line, and we are all so weak, you see, and we can slip so easily from being honestly happy about feeling better into thoughts of vanity, and competitiveness. And it occurred to me that one thing to keep an eye on as we continue to make progress would be our feelings about others making the same progress.

"I mean, if we're doing yoga because we want to inspire others to do it too, so they can heal themselves too, then if someone like the Sergeant began to do yoga, and suddenly got very good at it—able to do things we ourselves hadn't been able to do even after years of work—then I think our feelings about that would tell the story.

"I mean, if our motivation was pure, then we'd be excited and supportive: we'd let him know what a wonderful job he was doing. And if on the other hand we had started to slip into vanity, then I think we'd feel threatened somehow: we'd feel unhappy about his progress. And then that—that very basic, disappointing form of dislike for someone—would really start to choke our own channels, and ruin whatever progress we had been making. Do you see?"

"I do see," said the Captain frankly, "and I can tell you freely that my motivation, as always, was sort of mixed: a little hoping to inspire the men, and also hoping that they'd be impressed with me."

"I think all of us have that same problem," I mused. "And ultimately it's the cause for all the ups and downs in our lives . . . "

He opened his mouth to start to ask a question, but somehow I sensed that the right time for those particular ideas was still to come—perhaps soon.

"But what I really wanted to talk about today," I hurried on, "was an idea that lies behind that concept of focus. Because you'll be able to focus even better . . . "

"This yoga seems to unravel like an onion skin," laughed

the Captain. "Every time I think we've gotten to what lies at the bottom of everything else, you pull that layer off and show me another beneath it. Is there no one idea at the very bottom?"

And then when I answered "Later" he said it with me, like a chorus together, and we both laughed.

"Anyway, here's something to think about, when we're talking about focus, and how it affects your channels and inner winds. Normally, when someone tells us to focus, we have this picture in our minds of zeroing in on a thing, like a target.

"But if you really think about it, something else has to happen *before* the focus. I mean, you don't simply throw your attention out and hook the object you want to focus on, just like that. Rather, there's a process of elimination—like walking up into a large group of people, trying to find a friend of yours who's there. You don't just bump straight into him or her, usually. Usually it's a process: you work through the crowd of people, looking one way and then the other, *eliminating* groups and individuals as you narrow down the search for your friend; you arrive at where your friend *is*, really, by a process of weeding out where your friend *isn't*.

"And focus, you see, it's the same. Even just focusing on a smudge on the wall as you hold a yoga pose involves gaining some awareness of your other surroundings, and then *tuning them out* to arrive at your focus on the smudge.

"In the Master's *Short Book,* this process is called 'withdrawing the mind' from the outside world, to arrive at that clear, pin-point inner focus which is so helpful for clearing the inner channels. He says it like this:

Learn to withdraw the mind
From your physical senses;
Freed from its ties
To outer objects,
The mind can arrive
At its own real nature.

II.54

And there are a lot of levels also to withdrawing the mind from outer objects; to weeding out extra objects in order to arrive at the one we really want to focus on." I gazed around the room. "In fact, I can think of one very basic level right here, in front of us."

The Captain glanced around, so accustomed to his office that he literally didn't see what I was looking at.

"This place," I said, waving my arms around to the old stacks of papers; and the little piles of dirt everywhere; and cups and bowls of this and that lying atop any open surface. "This place is a *mess.*"

Again the Captain looked around, a little more slowly this time; but then his eyes came back to mine with that look that says, "Doesn't matter that much to me."

Out loud he said, "Does the fact that my office is, say, a little . . . cluttered . . . really have that much to do with my yoga?

"The Master seemed to think so," I responded. "Because he says,

The first commitment
Is to cleanliness.

II.32A"

The Captain looked unimpressed. But he had a good mind, and he wasn't afraid to think things out, and so I knew it would work if I went through the whole explanation.

"It all goes back to working on the channels from the outside," I began.

"Knocking on the pipes," he smiled, tapping the desk with his knuckles.

"Right," I said. "And so, so far we've talked about a number of things you can do from the outside of your body which go down and affect the subtle winds on the inside: things like the yoga poses themselves, and breathing in a very smooth and conscious way.

"And there's this constant interchange going on, you see; this constant interplay of the forces outside and inside of you. You get frantic at work often enough, and it ties up the inner channels. That causes an injury like your back: actually just a reflection of something going on deeper, in the channels. That makes you grumpy, which tightens the choke-points more, and then because you don't feel well you're not as careful about things in general. And one of those things is, well, just simple neatness: tidiness. A lack of this very basic kind of cleanliness—plain old tidiness—is almost a sure sign that your channels are 'untidy' too, deep down inside: the thought-winds are jumbled up, ready to turn into a new choke-point any time.

"And so a very simple and effective way to take advantage of the interchange, the interplay, between outside and inside is just to . . . " I waved my arms around again " . . . clean the place up! If where you live; if where you work; and especially if the place where you do your yoga poses is clean and tidy, then this is all reflected back upon the inner winds, . . . " I paused.

"And the channels loosen up, and the poses work even better on fixing you; on keeping you strong and healthy," finished the Captain.

"And you see, something else is at work here too. If there's just less junk around the room, then when you go to *focus*, and *fix* your mind on a single point, then there's not as many *things* that the mind has to sift through to get at what you want to focus on. It's a lot easier to find a friend in a group of ten people, especially if they are all lined up, than in a crowd of a hundred all milling around. Less effort, much less effort, to focus—all day long. Focus is like food for the mind: the mind thrives on it, and so do the good inner winds.

"And once you're done with your room," I said, "you can go further. I mean don't just tidy things up—*throw out* absolutely as many things as you can. Half the things that fill up our houses at any given moment are things that we *don't even use any more*, at all. And a good part of the other half is things that we rarely use, or don't really need to use anyway.

"And these extra things in our house, you see, they're tricky. I mean, it looks like they're just sitting there, pretty harmless, and that's why we let them stay there.

"But if I say, right now, 'Think of some of the things in your house' . . . " I paused again, so he could do it—and he got sort of an odd look on his face. "Then you can remember a great many things lying around your house, whether you ever use them or not. And that proves, you see, that they were taking up a part of your mind: you can remember them, because information about each one of them is stored in your mind. And the mind—although we don't often think of it this way—has only just so much capacity. Every time you acquire another object—every time there's one more thing cluttering up your home—then there's one more thing cluttering up your mind as well. And as the mind goes, so do the inner winds, and the choke-points in the channels."

"What you're saying, then," observed the Captain, "is that the more unused, use-less things I have lying around, the worse it is for my back, and even my peace of mind, because it hurts my channels."

"Just so," I said with a smile. "And when you're done clearing out the extra things around your house, then you have to go on to your very way of life and do the same. Throw out extra things you do that you really don't have time to do well, so you can focus. Throw out extra things you say that don't really need to be said anyway: learn to be with your friends, a few good friends, in a happy sort of silence that you both understand and appreciate. Cut down on all the extra, useless outside stimulation of your physical senses: too much food, too much news, too much 'entertainment,' too much physical gratification with the opposite sex; all of them fine in themselves, all of them healthy, but in moderation: in amounts that you can focus upon and enjoy deeply.

"And then the mind will be free to come inside, and arrive at its own nature: concentration, contemplation, uninterrupted attention—medicine for the channels, medicine for the inner winds, and so for health and a happy state of mind that lasts. It's all a kind of cleanliness, in a way: tidiness on the outside, tidiness on the inside."

The Captain nodded, but his eyes were fixed up somewhere over my head, and I knew his focus had wandered off. And then after a moment he snapped back.

"Well," he said, his voice shaking a bit, "I guess that means I'll have to get to work and tidy up my home, before . . . ah . . . "

"Before what?" I asked, completely unaware of where he was going.

"Well . . . ah . . . well, before you come to visit, next week," he smiled nervously. "For dinner," he added abruptly.

25

Two Invitations

Third Week of August

I was still feeling rather stunned by the Captain's invitation a full three days later, when the corporal came up to the bars of my cell and handed me through a package wrapped in a white cotton cloth and over-tied with string, the way a man would do it.

"Captain says, uh . . . let me see; he said to say it just so, and he made me practice it; Captain says, um . . . oh yes. Captain says you can wear this on Friday evening, but only if you really want to." Then the corporal blushed like a big boy, and turned and went to the side room, to hide for a while I think.

I stooped in the other back corner (the one without the hole) with my back to the front of the jail—which was my version of privacy—and I set the little package on my knees, and worked carefully at the knots. (*String*, you see, like all those normal little things you take for granted, is something important and valuable to a prisoner. *Time*, on the other hand, is not. And so I carefully undid all the knots, and carefully smoothed out all the string, before I even looked inside the package.)

It was an extraordinary piece of pale, sky-blue silk: the kind that an Indian woman would wrap around her on a holiday, along with one of those beautiful matching tops. That evening after dark I tried the whole thing on—it fit perfectly. It was not new, but it was very clean, and I felt the care for it and the goodness of the woman whose dress it had been. And as much as I understood how extra things can distract us from our higher selves, it felt good and right to be dressed in something fresh and beautiful, for going to the Captain's home. It felt to me that something important was going to happen there, and it deserved this special kind of cleanliness.

He had said to be ready by dusk on the appointed day; I dressed after doing my own daily yoga session, just before dawn, because that darkness was the last truly private moment I had every day. Then I wrapped my old ragged dress around the other, for the rest of the day, despite the heat.

I washed as well as I could with a cup of water in the afternoon, and then just waited around, well . . . nervously. And for some reason both the Sergeant and the corporal were standing around for hours too looking as nervous as little boys, and I could even feel Busuku being nervous in the next cell. I tried to sing the Master's *Short Book* in my mind, like I do whenever I have to pass some time like that, but I kept drifting off even before the end of the first chapter.

At what I figured was just about the moment before, I went into the back corner and got out the little dish with the last bit of the Sergeant's ointment in it. My wounds were almost completely healed, and what scars there were seemed to be fading. But the sandalwood scent of the oil always lingered.

And then he was there, dressed in a fresh white tunic with his red Captain's sash, and we went out in a surreal aura, to the second room on the side. It had a small low desk with several mats around it, and thick dust-covered ledgers stacked against the wall. The corporal stood around nervously near the door, while the Sergeant rummaged through the ledgers and finally pulled one out, and then the Captain said, "I want this done by the letter, Sergeant."

And the Sergeant looked up at him, and then over to me, but with a face so free of any unclean feeling that it struck me, like the fresh smell of the blue silk around me. And then he nodded, and turned to an open page, and made an entry noting that a prisoner was being escorted from the jail by the Captain on official business, and the Captain signed his name, and the corporal came and pressed his thumb in some ink and made the mark that was his signature, as an official witness.

And the Captain stood up very straight, and looked at his two men very sincerely, and said finally, "I am taking . . . my teacher, Miss Friday, to my home, because . . . " and there was a long pause. "Because I want to tell her . . . " he paused again, and looked into the Sergeant's eyes " . . . tell her about, about what happened, what happened . . . before. I think it will help . . . help, all of us. And the jail—it just, just doesn't feel like the place to say these things. Is it . . . is it clear? Do you . . . do you both see?" he asked. And they nodded as one, and we were gone—the Captain and I—out the front door, across the porch, to the path, to the road itself.

But there I paused, and glanced behind us, and the Captain smiled and said, "You are welcome to bring him too," and I ran back to the porch, where the Sergeant and the corporal were standing still gazing off at us like children left alone at home. The corporal was down the steps and back behind the building before I could say a thing, and brought out my little lion on the rope, and handed him over to me without a word.

People were out to walk in the evening cool and to buy their vegetables for dinner; a good number greeted the Captain formally on the road and stepped aside to stare at Long-Life and me, but all three of us were enjoying the air and the walk too much to notice them.

His house was a beautiful little white-washed bungalow standing by itself at the end of a road through some lovely green pastures. He showed me briefly around; it was simple: a small living room with a fireplace for cooking, and a tiny pantry off to the side; a pretty little room for bathing and toilet; and a quiet bedroom with lots of windows facing a green hill on one side and a small valley on the other.

He cooked and I watched, in silence, enjoying the nightfall and the feeling of my little precious one in my lap again. The Captain knew what he was doing with the food, and it told me a lot about his upbringing: subtle turns of spices, extra little stops along the way to let the savor set in. A well-off family, at least; but something else there too. He was a man who should have a fine wife, and children, and two or three servants doing all this cooking; but he had obviously chosen to live like this. I was intrigued.

We ate then too in silence together; it was not only that we really had only the one thing—the yoga—in common with each other, but it felt as well that each of us was collecting our thoughts, so we could speak of something of importance when the time came. And then it did, and he had poured us out cups of a wonderful sweet spiced tea, and he set everything else—neatly—to one side, and sat before me with an earnest look.

"There are things we need to speak of . . . ," he began, and there was no need to say more of it; we both knew.

"I will be frank with you," he said. "There are things I need to ask. I will go straight to the matter; we cannot stay too long." I nodded, happy with my little lion and the prospect of important words.

"You have fixed my back," he said, looking into my eyes with gratitude, "and if nothing else were said between us tonight, I would want to tell you how grateful I am. To be honest, I had simply expected to live with it that way, or worse, as I got older and older. And now I feel . . . I mean . . . not only has the pain gone, but I feel . . . I feel, somehow younger, somehow lighter than I have in many years—not only physically, but here as well," and he laid his hand over his heart.

I nodded again, sincerely, to thank him for his thanks. Gratitude too is one of the most powerful ways to free the middle channel. And then he looked out the back door, out over a beautiful little covered porch, for a long silent while. Then he came back to me, with his face set in a longtime sadness.

"But you see . . . there's something; there's something very obvious I need to ask . . . about this yoga. Perhaps it is . . . perhaps it is so obvious, that people forget to ask it, I think."

I nodded, and felt what was coming. His instincts really were so pure.

"You see, I know you have fixed my back—fixed my back and part of my heart, with the yoga. But I can't stop thinking—I can't help thinking—about what it really means in the long run.

"I mean, let's face it—let's be honest. In the end, really, it doesn't matter so much that my back is better. I mean—you and I know it—I will just keep getting older anyway, no matter how the yoga poses may help in their way to delay it, or help me make the best of what I have left as I grow older and older. But sooner or later something else will get hurt; sooner or later something else will fail; sooner or later, no matter how much energy the yoga gives me, my total level of energy will drop —is dropping, even as we speak—year by year; and then one day, and you and I both know it, and no matter how disciplined or determined I may be—well, one day, I will stop the yoga, because I just won't be able physically to do it any more, and then . . . and then . . . I will die, as all of us must die, and I'm not sure . . . I'm not sure then what the yoga, what doing the yoga, will have meant to me. It seems . . . it almost seems as though . . . it will have been, you see, almost fruitless, by the end, you see . . . " and he paused, and looked at the ground, and I knew he wanted to say something more; to tell me something.

"It's not that I'm not grateful, you see," he said finally, almost in apology, "but . . . but there are reasons why I ask this thing. There are reasons, good reasons—reasons I cannot escape—for asking you about these things." And with that finally he stood, and he went to the mantelpiece over the fireplace, and brought down a folder made with lacquered wooden covers. He opened it and handed it to me.

Inside there was a single piece of yellowed paper; a drawing, a portrait. It was a girl, a girl with long beautiful black hair, and eyes curving gracefully up, like the eyes of a Tibetan woman. Like . . . very much like, I realized, my own eyes. And then something began to dawn on me, and I looked up at him suddenly.

"I did not want to marry, you see," he began, his voice choked with emotion. And then it poured out of him. "I wanted . . . I wanted to stay with Uncle, you see. He was everything to me. We lived further north—north of here, you see—where the hills begin beneath the mountains, the mountains that connect your people's land to ours: the Himalayas.

"And Uncle, you see, he was different. You had to walk a long way across the face of the highest of the hills just to reach his house—his little hut, a stone hut. And you see, he was there—he lived there alone—so he could do, so he could do his yoga, you see, like you . . . and he did it the old way, like you are showing me, you see . . . not just the poses by themselves, but with the sitting, silently, and with . . . with the Master's *Short Book*, you see? The very same book. And he began to show me things like you do, with the breathing, and the focus, and he even began to teach me the letters of the Mother Tongue, of Sanskrit, you see . . . and . . . and that is how I could read, could read, just the cover . . . of your book, you see; and that is how . . . how I understand, how I feel, what you say, when you say it . . .

"But Father you see," and the sadness grew deeper in his face, "Father was afraid; Father was so proud of me, so proud to have a son at last, and so afraid when he saw how close I was growing to Uncle—to Uncle, who . . . who did . . . who it seemed, did nothing with his life—although, even then, you see, I knew, I felt—that it was only Uncle who was *not* doing nothing with his life."

He paused, remembering, almost unaware any longer of my presence. He looked into his tea and sipped it without thinking and went on. "So Father, you see—he arranged the marriage, as early as he could—and, and we married. And then, to make sure, he sent us away to the capital—he found me a job in the court, you see, in the King's court, you see.

"And those were the days of trouble, and the days of opportunity, you see. It was just three years after the old

King had died, and there had been a terrible struggle afterwards, and some noblemen had taken power, you see, done something—something to the Queen Mother, and to the Crown Prince, the older prince, you see—killed them, or sent them off into slavery, some say, in the Western Lands.

"But the year Father sent me to the court was the beginning of the New Realm, you see; the younger prince, who had escaped, he returned—returned with a strong army of his father's old allies. And they put him back on the throne, but they couldn't stay nearby forever, and it was a difficult time for the new King, you see, and he needed good people, new people, and my Father—he got me in.

"He got me into the ministry, you see—the Ministry of Justice—and I, I could read, and I could write, you see, our local language; and I worked hard, and within a year the Superintendent, you see—the same one who is Superintendent now, the one in charge of us—he noticed me, and he brought me up, close to him. And he was close to the new King, you see, because he had been very close to the old one: they had studied together—some of the things that Uncle had studied, and even with the same teachers—and that is how I was able to come to the capital, and begin my rise at court.

"And she was beautiful, as you can see, and she was good, and she respected the deeper things, you see—the things that Uncle had taught me to care about. And we set up our home in the capital there, you see, and it was a beautiful home—a home of simplicity and grace and hope—and near the end of that first year, we . . . we conceived a child, you see, and all our hopes—they were being filled there, before our very eyes."

He stopped abruptly, and looked down quickly at the floor, and his face suddenly twisted into itself and tears sprang down his cheeks. "And when it came time . . . time for the child . . . to be born, well, she labored—she fought, she screamed, she bled—to give it life. But in the end . . . at the end, it was born—our girl, she was born . . . born . . . dead, and . . . and the effort . . . to give her that . . . birth of death . . . it . . . it killed her too, you see? And I . . . I was left . . . left alone, with . . . with two dead bodies, and that . . . beautiful . . . home . . . of hope . . . " And he stayed there weeping, weeping without moving, for a long time. And Long-Life felt it too, the way he does feel things, deeply, and he got up out of my lap, and went and put his head on the Captain's knee. And without thinking the Captain stroked his fur, and in a while he was able to go on.

"And that was when . . . when I began to drink, you see, because it hurt so much, and nothing meant anything to me any more. And at first I would come to work late, and then I began to miss days, more and more days, because it felt like really there was not a lot of reason to get up out of bed in the morning. And then finally I began to drink in the daytime too, even in the morning, and I came to the office like that.

"And the Superintendent . . . he tried, he really did—he was so close to Uncle in his way of thinking, and such a generous man anyway, and he cajoled and covered and finally punished me however he could think of to get me out of it, but it was hopeless. And he and the young King, you see—they still had enemies, still have enemies even now, in the court and in the Ministry: people who would like any excuse to be rid of them. So in the end he had no choice, and he sent me here, to this godforsaken little town on the border—I have no idea why this one in particular, except that it was so forgotten by everyone that whatever other mistakes I made while I was drinking myself to death would go unnoticed.

"And Ravi was here—the Sergeant—and he was a good man; is still a good man. And those were good days, you see, at the beginning. Ravi took me in and got me excited about cleaning up the gangs of hoodlums that were terrorizing the lives of the people of this town all day long; and clean them up we did. Those swords and pikes on the wall at the station were not always rusted and dusty, you see: we fought hard, and we drank hard . . . ," and here he stopped again, and stared sadly at the floor.

"And Ravi, you see . . . Ravi, he didn't drink, before I came, you see . . . he was a good man, a family man, and a good officer—and then, it was *me*, you see, it was *me* who started him drinking—first for fun, to celebrate the thrill of the danger, and our victories, and then later for boredom, and then later . . . later on . . . for the sheer pain he was in, because of . . . " and here the Captain stopped cold, and wouldn't allow himself to go on with it. We were silent again, and he rubbed Long-Life's ears absent-mindedly.

"And then when that last thing happened, you see, I stopped—I had to stop, knowing I had been the cause of it all—but he . . . he couldn't, because the pain was always there, right in front of him. And he . . . he still stops, from time to time, but then the pain comes back on him hard for some reason, and it starts again. And even then, you see . . . " He stopped dead again, and looked me hard in the eyes.

"Even then, you see; even if our dream came true—even if all the silent sitting and seeing myself taking away his pain, and his drinking—even if it worked, you see; even if it came true—and even if giving him the most precious thing I have left in my life could really happen; even if somehow he became Captain, well you see . . . even then, I'm not sure, deep inside me, what it would all mean, what it would mean in the end, you see," and he placed his hand sadly on his wife's likeness, "if it all has to fall apart again anyway: if a sober and successful Sergeant, or Captain, has to go through the degradation, and humiliation, and travesty of that gradual fall into old age, and weakness, and the loss of all we hold dear—and then death itself—regardless of whether we ever did yoga or not. What would it mean?" he pleaded. "What does it mean?"

My instincts told me to stay silent; there was still something there in him, to come. And again he lifted his eyes past me and stared out the door, past the porch, into the dark. Then they came back to mine, strong and clear now.

"I said I wanted to speak honestly, to speak openly with you. And I have. But there is . . . there is one more thing," he said with a powerful kind of strength now.

"You see Uncle, when I was young, just a boy really, he didn't just teach me the beginning yoga poses, and some exercises with the breath, and focus and letters and all that. Sometimes, sometimes, when we were sitting there, like this, in the evening, alone, over a warm cup of tea—his root tea, you see—then he would look out into the dark of the sky that stretched over the plains beneath us—over all of Mother India, before us, you see—and he would talk about wonderful things, about . . . " and the Captain paused a bit, seeming almost embarrassed, " . . . about, you see, people who had learned all of the yoga, the deeper yoga—the yoga of the Master's *Short Book*. And Uncle said, you see, he said that . . . if you had a good teacher, and you really tried with all your heart, then you could . . . you could, you see, go to heaven, you see—I mean, what they always talk about, it could really happen to you, to anybody at all, no matter what your age or whether you were man or woman, rich or poor, successful or not—you could, you could really one day meet . . . Angels, beautiful, holy creatures, and you could . . . learn to be with them, learn to stay with them, and you would even yourself change, change one day . . . and be like them, made of pure light, passing through every realm of living things, man and beast, constantly helping them, constantly nurturing them, like your own children, and then . . . and then, one day make them like you—angelic, indestructible light, perfect love, spreading to every living creature in need, and curing them.

"And I was young then, too young, and I bore the curse of youth—I had health, I had strength, I had not seen death and tragedy, I was sure I was immune to them in any event—and I simply didn't hear what he was saying. But the seed, you see . . . the seed was planted, then; a vision of what could really be, a vision of what the word 'yoga' really means—a *union* with things divine.

"And the seed stayed in me, within me, all that time, and then—when you . . . when you came to me . . . and you . . . you looked so much like her . . . her or perhaps our daughter, and exactly the age she would have been; but either way like an Angel, the way I know an Angel would look to me—like them—and then, when we opened the Master's book, and you read that line, that line about how we think things will last, when they never do . . . well in that moment, the seed broke open in me, you see, and hope came in me . . . hope, to hope for the things . . . the things that Uncle spoke about. Because he said too that . . . that when the Angels came—as we began to reach them, as we begin to *become* them, then . . . all the ones we love, too . . . all the ones we have ever loved, and ever will love, you see, he said . . . they come. He said, they all come. He said, they come, and we are together, and that . . . this was real yoga; this was the real reason for every part of yoga, whether it is the yoga poses, or the breathing, or the focus, or the sitting.

"And all I ask you tonight here is, is it possible? Can it really work that way? Can we go beyond death, and old age, like this? Is it a way to heaven? Is there a heaven? Can we meet Angels? Are there Angels? Can we . . . become like them, light and pure love? Can we learn to make others that way too? And will we . . . will we all, be . . . be, in the end . . . together, like that? Do you know these things? Can you . . . " and then his voice broke into a sob, and his head came down nearly to the floor, before me, "can you . . . will you . . . teach me, teach us these things?"

A power came into me, a power like the power that Katrin had, and I put my hand on his head, and held it there softly, warmly, touching the seed in him, making the hope grow real. And I gave him silence, so he could feel it, and never forget it.

And then I said, softly, "All the things your Uncle said, all those things . . . they are true. The Master too, he says,

> *And there will come a time*
> *When they invite you*
> *To take your place with them.*
>   III.52A"

He looked up, quiet now, and I looked down at him. "You are invited," I said gently, with words that were not my own. "And now the real work begins."

26

Flesh or Light

Fourth Week of August

At our next class the Captain fairly dragged me to his room; he was excited as a little boy, a far cry from the tired, grumpy office worker I had met on the first day.

"Questions!" he exclaimed. "Lots of questions! I've been thinking about *everything*!"

Then he stopped suddenly and looked at me with a touch of worry in his face. "But something else . . . first. Something else we have to talk about."

I nodded simply, and he went on.

"You see, wherever we go from here . . . I have to say first, I have to admit, that you have . . . you have cured my back, and you obviously know what you are doing with the yoga, especially with yoga in the broader sense—from channels to breath to mind and heart, and further . . . " He looked up with anticipation.

"And so really, I know . . . we both know, that the book really is yours, and that you cannot have stolen it, regardless of what the Sergeant said all along . . . ," and then he paused.

I raised an eyebrow. "Said . . . all along?" I asked.

The Captain reached out and toyed with the . . . pen . . . on his desk a little nervously, and then said, with a slightly puzzled look on his face, "Yes, you see . . . the Sergeant, well—I mean, didn't you ever wonder, wonder *why* he was out in that little guardhouse at the checkpoint on the day you came through? I mean, have you ever seen him, or the corporal, ever go out to man that crossing gate again, during the whole time you've been here?"

And then it dawned on me what he was saying. No, I hadn't wondered, and I really should have. I looked back at the Captain, puzzled now myself.

"Well it was about a week before that, you see, and the Sergeant, he comes to me and he tells me that he's gotten word—word from some informant, some unnamed informant—that a girl matching your description, a foreigner, from Tibet, accompanied by a dog matching *his* description," and the Captain waved in Long-Life's general direction, "is going to be attempting to cross into the borders of the Realm carrying contraband—some kind of stolen articles—and that we should post a guard there, on that particular road, to intercept her."

My mouth dropped full open now. I tried to remember if I had met anyone on the road, before that, who could possibly have gotten such an idea, and sent word ahead.

"And so," the Captain was speeding on, "and so, you can't really blame us—blame me—for being so careful with you. But now, of course—now it is all so obvious—so obviously just a very terrible error of some kind, and you really should be released."

I sat back a little stunned, and he glanced up and then down again, and hurried on. "Except that, you see . . . you see, we really *can't* release you now."

His eyes came up again, but I didn't really feel much either way, to tell you the truth. My thoughts were elsewhere: on the class, on the place we would start from today.

"Don't you want to know why not?" he exclaimed.

"Sure, all right, yes . . . please," I said, coming back to myself.

"Well, you see, on the day that you tried to escape . . ." I shot him a fiery glance. "Er . . . I should say, on the day that it *seemed* you had tried to escape, I wrote a report . . . I was required to write a report, you see, informing the Ministry that we had in custody a foreigner who had attempted to escape. And now, you see, you are on record, and the Ministry people—they are especially careful with foreigners, given the delicate situation between the King and the various other factions. There is no way I could release you now—no way I could report it as a simple mistake—without causing a lot of trouble, and accusations aimed at the Superintendent by his enemies in the Ministry, who would see any correspondence I sent in. And so, we will have to wait."

"Wait? For what?" I asked.

"For the Superintendent himself to come, you see, and then I can explain everything in person, with no correspondence. As I told you, he received some training in the ways of yoga as far back as the times of the old King— who at one point even had an illustrious teacher of yoga advising him. The Superintendent will understand; he will give us approval to release you, and then he'll be able to deal with the people in the Ministry when he returns."

"So, when will the Superintendent be here?" I asked— but strangely I was more engrossed in thinking about how to guide the Captain through the pathway of ideas just ahead of him.

"Uh . . . that's a bit of a problem, you see," he replied.

"The Superintendent—well, he makes it a point to visit every facility like this in the Realm at least once a year . . . "

The *once a year* struck me, and suddenly it sounded to me that I should perhaps listen to what the Captain was saying.

"Or . . . or so," continued the Captain, who had at least mastered official vagueness during his time in the capital. "You see," he explained, "it is frankly dangerous for the Superintendent to announce the itinerary for his visits, since the countryside roads would be a perfect place for people of the different factions to ambush him. He is also a very strict and dedicated leader, as was the old King, his friend. He demands regular reports of all our border skirmishes and such, and he likes his visits to be a surprise, so he can really see how we work from day to day."

"All your . . . border skirmishes?" I asked, and here the Captain reddened a bit. Then he sat up straight and gestured to the piles of reports stacked around him.

"The people in the Ministry—not the Superintendent, you see, but many of the people who work around him, people who would like to see him and his ideas thrown out, along with the young King—they would never allow this station to exist, if they didn't think we were actively holding off constant incursions from the other side of the border. And if this station didn't exist, then the gangs would be back hurting the people here within a few weeks, and all the work we have done to make them safe would be lost, forever. And so . . . and so . . . you see, I make up the skirmishes, and then I write the reports, and then . . . you see . . . it keeps the common people of this town safe; something that the factions so influential in the Ministry couldn't care less about."

Suddenly I grasped something, something important—and then the Captain's path to what he really dreamed of, his path to the dream his Uncle had given him, came clear.

"Ah," I said, beginning him down the path. "So now I see," I said, waving to the stacks of reports. The Captain looked puzzled.

"You see . . . why, why you may have to stay inside this jail for months and months; maybe *many* months more?" he asked.

"Inside?" I replied, distractedly. "Why, oh, whatever. Of course I have to stay here. We decided that when we spoke at your house, or before," I said flatly. "But no, that's not what I mean. I mean that now I see, I see how your back was cured."

"My back?" he asked, reaching around instinctively to where he had held it all those years. "Why, it was the yoga, of course . . . the exercises, and I'm sure the silent sitting and good wishes for the men helped—I mean, you know, loosening the choke-point and all that; knocking on the pipe from the outside; cleaning it out from the inside—inner winds, and all that, you see. I *know* why my back got better."

I shook my head. "That's not *why* your back got better," I said with finality, "that's just *how* your back got better. What I just understood was *why* your back got better. And until you understand *why* your back got better, you won't even understand really *how* your back got better, either."

He looked at me a little confused. That was all right. Learning these things takes some time—some time to get all the explanations, some time to ask your questions, some more time to get them answered. And now we would start.

"I mean," I said, "it's something we began to talk about a long time ago. Lots of people have aches and pains—things

that come to us all, more and more, the older we get." He
nodded.

"And people try different things to stop the aches and
pains—and a certain number of people end up trying yoga:
the yoga exercises, the poses. And you see—let's put it
bluntly. The yoga works for some of them, and it doesn't
work for others. And even with the people it works for, it
stops working at some point, as they get older. And then
they just get older and older, and eventually they die, like
everyone else. We said all this before."

"But the channels," he objected. "The inner winds: you
explained everything. Yoga works for you if you know how
to use it on the channels, on the choke-points, from the
outside and the inside."

"Not enough," I said. "Not enough. We have to go
deeper."

He gave me a look that said he didn't really *want* to go
deeper. He felt all right today, and going deeper—it was an
effort, an effort that we all avoid, in our own way, until life
forces us forward. Or unless we have a teacher to drag us
there.

"Think!" I said finally. "Think! You have to think about
it! Now it's not just the Sergeant, and the corporal, and you
know it! Now it is—now it is the wonderful woman whose
blue dress I wore that night; now it is the daughter you
made with her, together. It's time to ask, time to find out.
It's not fair to them, it's not fair to ourselves, to just go on
quietly with what little we understand, incomplete, until
it's too late for us to help ourselves or anyone else!

"What *made* the channels?

"What put the winds inside of them?

"Why does a wind decide to turn one way, and not
another? Why do we decide to turn one way, and not
another, at every fork in the road of our lives?

"What really brought you to this town? What brought me here? Why have we met? Why did you hurt your back—not *how*, at this particular little desk—and why, why did it get better?

"And could we go further—could we change your body altogether? Does it need to be this way? It is all the questions you asked me the other night—and now we need to answer them, and you have to follow me, and think hard, and work hard. There are so many lives at stake; so many, if what your uncle said was true. Do you see? We need to ask, and we need to work, hard. It doesn't matter that we are inside a jail. Everyone is inside a jail. We need to get out . . . to get out of the bigger jail: this entire life, this life that always leads to death and ruin."

He looked up at me, with hope, but then he shook his head. "You gave me hope; you give me hope, every time you speak like this. But then when I am alone again, I start to think. And the first thought that comes to me is always the same, always the same, and it always stops all the other thoughts that might have come after it."

I waited for the question that I knew was coming. A person who didn't think to ask it first was not a worthy vessel for the knowledge the Captain sought: the knowledge of life itself.

"You see," he said, "you can talk of deeper causes; you can talk of how the body really works, and you can talk about some miraculous method of changing it at these deepest levels; you can even talk—quietly, in the stillness of our most private thoughts—about changing this body forever, of going as light itself to live in a place of light among beings who are pure light and love themselves." He paused, to calm himself, and gazed for a moment out the window.

"But whatever you say—however inspiring your words might sound, in the moment—one cold fact remains, and it kills your words: it has always killed those words for me, and always will, until I learn better.

"What I mean to say is," he uttered finally, "is that—aside from stories, and myths, and old tales we hear repeated now and again, never anything that you could prove, never anything that you can actually *see*—well, no one that we can meet face to face has ever really changed like that, like what you spoke about. I mean, no one that we can actually see has ever used the wonderful methods you speak of, to change: to change into light, to go to a place of perfect and never-ending happiness, and to . . . to stay there with . . . with the ones they love, with . . . with the ones they loved, as you . . . as you, and Uncle . . . claimed we could do." And then he closed his mouth into a thin tight sad line, and stared at me, almost in accusation.

And it is the first question, and it should be the first question. And I had taught him the answer already—he knew it already—but it was just too immense really to keep his mind on for that long.

"The Master says," I began, "that we must

> *Stay in that one pure thought,*
> *And never forget it;*
> *That single most important thing:*
> *Things are empty*
> *Of being what they are*
> *By themselves.*
>
> I.43A"

He shook his head tightly, forcefully. He almost saw, and he didn't see, and it was killing him. I picked the pen up from his desk, and held it up between us—my shining golden sword.

"Is this a pen; or is it something to eat?" I demanded.

He shook his head again, violently. Help me.

I leaned over intensely and slammed my palm into his chest.

"Is this flesh—born only to die; or is it pure and loving light?"

He looked up at me, his face changing.

"And your wife, and your daughter," I said, loudly now, thrusting my palm there, at his chest, where the highest compassion of all lies choked. "Are they dead, and gone forever; or do they stand at your side, waiting to be seen, waiting until you *learn to see them, be with them, be them?*"

And then I slammed my hand down again on the desk and held the pen up between us. "Is it a pen, or something to eat? *Answer me!*" I screamed.

"A pen!" he screamed back now, nearly across the border. "A pen!"

"No!" I screamed back. "Not a pen! Never a pen! *Never a pen!* No cow has ever seen this pen, as a pen, and so . . . " I waited for him.

"And so, and so . . . they would say . . . cows would say . . . that there are no pens," he finished, still thinking it out.

"The mind makes it a pen," he went on to himself. "It is not a pen . . . by itself. It is empty of that . . . by itself."

And then he looked down, at his own chest, where my hand had woken him. "And the body . . . my body, this flesh . . . " he said, holding his own two hands there, with a look of wonder growing on his face. "It is flesh, it is flesh, because . . . because . . . and *only* because, my mind makes me see it that way."

Then his chin jolted upright and his eyes burned into mine.

"But how . . . how to *change* it?" he breathed.

And I nodded at his understanding and said, "It is what I have to teach you now."

27

Seeds, and
Not Decisions

First Week of September

"When we stop and think carefully about this pen," I began, rolling it in my fingers, "then it's very clear that what is—its *pen*-ness—is not coming from itself, from its side. That much, if we are just honest with ourselves and think carefully for a few moments, is obvious. Because . . ." I let him finish it.

"Because if it *were* a pen by itself, from its *own* side, then every creature who ever came in contact with it would see it as a pen. It would, in a sense, be shouting out 'pen' to every being that ever looked at it. But it doesn't act that way, announcing itself like that, say to a cow, or to a fly that lands on it," concluded the Captain, eloquently.

"Correct," I said. "But the fact is that us people do see this . . . this green stick . . . as a pen, don't we? And if that's not coming from its side, then it must be coming from . . . "

"From *our* side," he finished, almost impatiently. "Where *else* could it come from? It *has* to be our own minds that make us see this green stick as a pen; and it must be the cow's mind making *her* see the *same* green stick as, well . . . as just something good to eat." And then he looked frustrated, as if he were about to burst, and I waited for the question I knew was coming.

"But there's a *problem* with that," he blurted out. "Because it *can't* be, you see, that it's just my mind making me see it as a pen!"

"And why not?" I said, cold as steel, the way Katrin would have said it.

"Well, it's obvious," he steamed on. "Completely obvious. If it really were just my mind making me see this as a pen well then I could just *decide* to see it any way I wanted, you see. Like I could just *decide* to see this green stick as a bar of gold, and that's what it would be, if it were just *my own mind* making me see it as a pen."

I nodded. This was the usual way a person's thinking would flow, once they started to get the idea.

"Well the Master answers that very question, in the *Short Book*. He says,

Countless seeds within our minds
Make us see
The great variety of things around us.

IV.24A

The point is," I explained, "that we don't have any *choice* about how our minds make us see something. Because they *force* us to see it that way. Because our minds, you see, are full of millions and millions of tiny seeds. And as we look at something, some of those old seeds—seeds that were planted there before—well they ripen, and they make us see the thing as we do: *force* us to see the thing as we do. And so it *is* our minds that make us see a thing the way we do, but it's not at all that we are controlling the process as it happens.

"And I think it might help you here if we say a little bit more about how it all happens, because it happens so fast—all in just one moment, always in the one fleeting present moment. The Master goes on to explain it like this:

> *The way it works*
> *Is that they organize*
> *Other parts in a certain way.*
>
> IV.24B

You see, there are always some other parts involved. Let's take the pen. In this case, the 'other parts' are a cylindrical shape, and some green color. In fact, if you think clearly about it, this is another indication that it's *your* mind that's making you see the pen as a pen."

The Captain cocked his eye at the pen, trying to thresh it out, and I guided him ahead swiftly.

"You see, if you really think about it, our eyes—our sense of sight—work in a very limited little world: that is, in shapes and colors. Your *eyes*, as such, can only detect shapes and colors. And once they *have* detected shape and color—in our case, a cylindrical shape and some green color—then their only job is to pass this information along to the mind. And then the mind thinks about it, and organizes all this data into an object—into a thing.

"Now which thing it decides to organize out of these other parts is *not* up to us, you see, or things would always just be what we wanted them to be; and the hard facts of life inform us quite clearly that this is not the way it works.

"No, it's different: something else is at work; something behind the scenes, something outside of our conscious control. And this power behind the scenes is the seeds within our minds: countless seeds. *They* decide how our mind goes

183

ahead and organizes these other parts into a thing. A cow's mind has seeds that ripen in that moment and organize the reports of colors and shapes into the image of a tasty little morsel. *Our* minds have *different* seeds that ripen at the very same moment, but which organize the same colors and shapes into a pen.

"And why does the Master say 'countless' seeds? Why, look around you; gaze upon the incredible variety of things around you at any given moment, and all their details. *Every little detail* of the things you see around you has to be an image, a *separate* image, organized by the mind—which is forced to do so as more seeds ripen to organize each detail into itself.

"And that's just the things we can *see*," I pushed on. "But everything else we can ever be aware of—outside us, inside us, inside our own thoughts, and memories, hopes, ideas, dreams—they are all the same. All of them images, all of them things, sketched into being from other parts, other pieces put together as the seeds within our minds force our minds to put them together.

"And all *real*, you see?" I wanted to make sure right away that he didn't fall into that common trap. "All *real*, you see? All *working*, really *working*, as the objects we see them to be. The pen is an object that the seeds in our minds force our minds to piece together, yes, but the pen *works*, you see? It's *real*, it *works*; and that's exactly *why it works*. And the same for . . . "

"For something nice to eat," he finished with a smile. "It may be true . . . well, I guess it *has* to be true . . . that it is only the *seeds* in the cow's mind making it see this same green cylinder as a snack. But that doesn't make it any less real, or tasty, or solid in the cow's stomach. In fact, if I understand

184

you right, it explains exactly *why* this cylinder can fill the cow's stomach."

"Beautiful," I whispered in hushed tones. "Beautiful. You got it."

He leaned over the desk at me, happy, and with every reason to be happy. "No, I *didn't* get it," he whispered back, with a smile.

I frowned back. "Didn't get what?"

"Didn't get . . . where the *seeds* come from!"

"Ah that," I said.

"Later!" we chorused.

"Time to knock on the pipes!" I added.

"I was hoping you'd forgotten," he said, his face already dripping from the summer heat. "Can't we just concentrate on cleaning the pipes from the inside? Isn't it much more powerful?" he asked.

"It is," I agreed. "But working from the outside—the yoga poses, the special ways of breathing—it's something so concrete, something anyone, anywhere, at any age, in any frame of mind, can roll up their sleeves and get their bare hands on, and make gradual, steady, measurable progress on from day to day. And that in itself is powerful . . . unspeakably powerful. We need things like that. They go together—a perfect union, yoga, inside and out."

"All right," he said with resignation, and stood up to sweat some more.

28

Seeds are Planted

The next class we went straight to the point. It's best to do very important things as soon as you can, because the more important they are, the better the chances that something might happen to stop them. And this certainly turned out to be a day like that.

"So let's summarize where we are so far," I began. "It's not the case that we see the pen as itself—as a pen—because it's a pen from its own side. Otherwise Mrs. Cow might have tried to write a letter with it—but she didn't. So it must be something in our own minds that makes us see it as a pen. And last week we saw that *how* our minds organize things into things is not just something we can consciously decide: otherwise we wouldn't have any of the problems in life that we do have, since we could just wish things into things we wanted.

"And so there must be other forces at work, behind the scenes: forces beyond our current control. And the Master said that these forces are seeds; certain seeds in our minds, ripening moment by moment and forcing our minds to organize bits and pieces of information into images — into things themselves."

"Small problem, right there," interjected the Captain, raising his hand, almost like a boy in a classroom. I knew what his problem was, but I let him go ahead and say it. He was *such* a wonderful student. He actually *took things home* and *thought* about them, over and over, until he came to the next logical question with them.

"What's that?" I said, playing along.

"I understand that there may be seeds in my mind that step into the act when I look at some cylinder-shaped patch of green, and make me see it as a pen. But what about . . . "

"The green itself?" I said. "You tell me. There are people who can't see colors, you know: color-blind people. Same thing. No seeds. They don't have any seeds going off in their mind and organizing the *other parts* into a patch of color. And in this case the *other parts* are the left side of the patch, and the right side of the patch. Even colors and shapes are still just images pieced together by our minds . . . " I paused.

"Forced to do so, by the seeds there—the seeds in each separate person's mind," he concluded. "But then why," he blurted.

"Why do we see the same objects? Why do you and I both see this thing as a pen, if the pen isn't coming from its own side? You tell me," I challenged him.

He frowned and thought for a moment. "Same . . . same seeds? Same kinds of seeds?" he asked.

"Exactly," I said, "or nearly so. Of course the two of us see—and that's *why* we see—the same pen in a slightly different way. But insofar as we both see a *pen* at all, well— we have the same kinds of seeds in our two minds."

"But now you must do as you promised," he said seriously, "and tell me—where do the seeds come from, in the first place?"

"Because . . . ," I prompted him.

"Because," he said, gazing at something outside the window, something beyond the sky. "Because, because if what we've said is true—if we are seeing this thing as a pen only because there are seeds in our minds that force us to see it as a pen—then . . . then if we could *change* the seeds; if we could *affect* these seeds; if we could cultivate certain seeds purposely, and destroy undesirable seeds; then I don't see any reason why we couldn't eventually see . . . see . . . "

"Say it," I said.

"See ourselves, see our very own bodies, flesh and blood, turn into light; sort of the ultimate yoga pose, if you think about it. And then as well we could . . . we could turn this process further, on the things around us. I mean, theoretically, if what we have said is true—and I see no reason why it should *not* be true—then we really could come to a place of perfect light, as light ourselves, and be with . . . be with all those with whom we have suffered so far through this life, all of us the same—the same . . . light."

"Perfect," I breathed again. "And so we must understand how the seeds work, and again this is all part of the deeper yoga that the Master has passed on to us so perfectly. And here he says,

> *The storehouse is planted*
> *By the things we do.*
>
> II.12B

When he says 'storehouse' here, the Master is talking about the storehouse in our own minds: the place where the seeds stay, until they ripen and compel our minds to organize other parts into an image, into a thing.

"And he answers that most important question—he tells us where the seeds come from—by saying that they are 'planted by the things we do.' And if you think about it, it makes sense on a very basic level. *Something* has to have put all these seeds in our minds, and this is obviously not the kind of thing where someone can come along and get say a handful of beans into your mind by pouring them into one of your ears. If the seeds ripen as perceptions—as something mental—then it makes sense that they were planted by mental perceptions in the first place. And what the Master is saying is that we plant these seeds every time as we perceive ourselves *do* something: *anything.*"

The Captain made that frown of his again, and then said, "But anytime we do something—whenever we do *anything*—well of course we perceive ourselves doing it: we see ourselves doing it, on some level or another."

"Exactly so," I said, "and so *everything* we ever do—any action we ever take; any word we ever utter; even the very *thoughts we think*—they all plant seeds in our minds, simply as we are aware, in any way, that *we are doing them.* Seeing ourselves do them plants a seed, makes an imprint on the mind, like pressing your hand into a lump of clay.

"And the actions, or the words, or the thoughts—they may stop, and we may go on to something else—but the imprint made on our minds, it stays there. And it becomes a seed, a seed that will determine how we see our world later on.

"And so now let's take a real example: let's say you're walking down the road out there and you see a man who said something unpleasant to you a few days before. And so you make up some excuse to hit him with your policeman's stick, on the back.

"In the very moment that you decide to hit him, a thought flashes through your mind: you have a picture, a vague picture perhaps, of him holding his back in pain just after you hit him. And then you do hit him; you see yourself actually doing it, and you see a much clearer image of his pain, with your own eyes. And then later perhaps on the way back to the station you think with satisfaction about how you got back at him for what he did: in your mind's eye you see yourself again, hitting him, and him in pain. Each time the pain is anticipated, or actually seen, or reflected upon later, well then an imprint is placed in your own mind: like a handprint left in soft clay.

"And this imprint, an imprint of pain you have caused in someone else's back, it stays there: it becomes a seed. And then one day, your mind goes to some *other parts* . . . " I paused to see if he could pick up the thread.

He hesitated, but then it came to him. "Other parts, say, like the bones in the lower part of my spine."

"And the seed ripens just then: the image of pain planted in the clay comes to the front of the mind, and . . . "

"And I am sitting at my desk, hunched over an important report in the middle of the eighth year of my service here, and suddenly I feel—I mean, my mind *makes* me feel—I mean . . . " He paused; he got it.

"I mean . . . the *seeds* in my mind, they ripen, and that imprint—that old image of pain, in the area of the back, that was planted *when I saw myself* cause *someone else* that pain— it comes back to me, to me myself, making me feel . . . the very same . . . *pain*," and his hand went instinctively to his back.

Then he stopped, and I could see the ideas begin to pour through his mind. And he said, excitedly now, "You know, it makes sense. I mean, you know, I'd always heard about this kind of idea—I mean, people all the time are talking about how what you do comes back to you—but I, but nobody really, we never take it seriously, because . . . well, because it wasn't very clear how it would all work, really. I mean, you think about it, and it seems to make sense—it would be a perfect kind of justice, in the entire universe, really—if what you did to others always came back to you; and if, looking at it the other way around, *everything that ever happens* to us *only* happens to us *because* we have done the same thing to someone else.

"But until you explained it to me the way you did—I mean, starting with the pen, you see, and the cow, and really proving to me beyond any argument that it must be something *in my own mind* that makes *me* see it as a pen— well, until then, this idea of a sort of inescapable justice on a grand scale was just something that sounded like it *should* exist, rather than something that *does* exist: something that *does* exist and dictates . . . well then, *every single detail of our lives*, every single detail of the world around us.

"It's so *pure*," he said, looking into my eyes with a kind of reverence, "and it's . . . it's so overwhelming!" He moved his hand up to his forehead and rubbed it the way he used to rub his bad back.

"A lot of questions . . . ," he said then.

"The more the better," I answered. "It's the only way to learn." But it still didn't get him out of his poses.

φ

That night I was fast asleep, and then a sound outside the bars of my cell woke me. I thought it was some terrible dream, some memory of what had happened before, but it was terribly real—and now. It was the Sergeant, again, hanging onto the bars with his hands, his eyes drunk and gleaming red, once again, and the stink of the liquor filling the late night air.

"You will come with me," he said, and without a question I knew he meant it, deadly serious this time. He had gotten another stick somewhere, and it crackled against the bamboo bars as he lifted the crossbar free of the door.

"Ravi, Ravi! What are you doing now?" came Busuku's sleepy voice.

"Shut up Busuku!" roared the Sergeant, and I heard the stick flail down the line of bars on the other side, and a sharp cry as it struck Busuku's knuckles. "Ravi!" he called again, in a warning of his own.

"Nothing to worry about this time anyway, Busuku. And I tell you the truth." The Sergeant stood tall, weaving, inside the cell now; and he said to the wall there, to the dead dusty wall, "Because . . . because . . . I am taking her . . . to see . . . to see the boy," he said simply, but with so much pain that it hurt my own heart to hear it.

Busuku went silent then, totally silent, and I felt that it meant I should go with the Sergeant.

And so I did, through the darkness, following the dark form, and the sound of the stick dragging useless on the ground, and the sickening smell of the liquor.

We went a fairly long way, out near the old woman's house, and then beyond. Up a small road, and into a small yard that spoke of ruin and neglect. Into a dark room where his smell had been so often so long that every article in the room seemed soaked in it. And there was a small fire in a small hearth, just for the light, and a small figure—a child—hunched before the flame in a blanket, with its back to us.

Near the door was a single bare table, with a single candle, and sitting on a mat behind it was a woman, an old woman. I studied her face in the silence: it was creased deeply with a lifetime's lines of pain, and little white scars around the eyes, and the lips—all framed in a shock of white hair. And then I suddenly realized that she was the Sergeant's wife, and I suddenly saw all the beatings she had lived through, and I saw in her eyes the undefeated kindness that so often grows within a person subjected to this worst and daily pain.

And she smiled softly, to say "Please excuse my husband," without saying it, and not saying it said to me that she would be beaten again if it were. And we understood each other fully in that first moment, and I nodded, and she nodded back ever so slightly. And then the Sergeant and I sat at the table, and the kind woman pushed me a little cup of warm simple tea, and the Sergeant pulled a clay jug from under the table, and took a deep long draught, and then fixed those angry crimson eyes on my own.

"I was drunk," he said, and he drank again. "Got drunk with the Captain, like we used to do." He paused, and drank again.

"I came home. They were sleeping. She and the boy." And he waved the jug towards the figure sitting before the fireplace. He lifted it to his lips again, but then simply set it down on the table.

"I . . . I . . . " He stared at me. His face twisted, and tears sprang out. "I . . . knocked over a candle, a candle . . . like this one," and he stared into the small flame, and jagged lines of tears inched down his face. The woman looked away.

"The straw, you see. They . . . we . . . were sleeping on some straw, you see. And it . . . it caught fire. And I . . . at first I didn't notice—too drunk to notice—and then they

193

are screaming, she and the boy are screaming, and the flames . . . the flames are up in my face, and I don't know what to do, I don't know what I am doing, but I tell myself, I say to myself, 'Ravi; you are an officer, an officer of the Realm. And you . . . you are trained, trained in the Royal Academy itself, and you . . . you know how to act, you know when to act, and so now, just carry out your duty, as you have been trained to do'; and I calm myself, and I reach into the flames, and I feel the two arms there, and I grab onto them with all my might, and I tear us from the fire, and from the house, kicking and screaming, and then outside I am wondering 'Why? Why kicking and screaming? Why still kicking and screaming?'

"And I look down into my hands, at the arms in my hands, my hands, closed like steel vices . . . and . . . and . . . " The woman cried in pain, despite herself.

"And . . . you see, it is only *her* two arms—I am holding on, only to *her* two arms—and then finally I can hear what she is screaming, and she is screaming 'The boy! The boy!'

"*Boy!*" he suddenly exploded. "*Boy!* Get up! Come here!"

And the little blanket at the fireside stirred, and stood slowly, stiffly, and the boy came to the table, and his face came to the light.

What I saw first was the kindness and softness in his eyes; love, as if he had never lived in this house, with this man turned demon—and as if he had never seen the reflection of his own face. And the face, the face, I saw then—it was slick and red on one side, as if it were wax, wax that had melted and fallen into his neck, glued there now in a web of angry skin. I started to cry, despite myself; not at his ruined face, but at the pain he must have had, and the pain he had now, underneath his obvious courage.

The Sergeant sat for a moment studying the same face, crying steadily. And he reached out and held what remained of the cheek, and said only "My boy," in a voice of love and pain.

And then he turned to me and said, "Can you fix him? Can you fix something . . . like this . . . like you fixed . . . like you fixed the Captain's back?"

The woman moaned at her husband's impossible hope. He didn't even hear.

"And his leg," he went on excitedly. "His leg, you see. Boy! Walk over to the fire, and back! Show her . . . show her your leg!"

And with unspeakable unfathomable cheerfulness the boy looked up into my eyes warmly and turned and dragged himself to the fire, one leg flopping weakly, and then back again. And he looked up again at me, not really hoping, but just because of the love in him, love for anyone. And Katrin came into me and I was sitting with the Captain holding up that glorious pen of truth between us and turned to the Sergeant and his wife and I said "Anything . . . anything is possible."

And then I am outside the doorway of that dark house again, but now the moon is out, and the Sergeant is looking into my face and I in his and I say, "But there is one condition."

"Anything," he says.

"You must come to learn as well. You must be cured as well."

He shook his head sadly. "The sickness I have cannot be cured. I stop, it stops, and then it always comes back. You cannot ask me for that. I cannot learn it, even from you."

I shook my head resolutely, in the dark. "You can learn, you must learn. And not from me."

He looked down at me, puzzled.

"You will learn . . . you will learn from the Captain."

He opened his mouth to object.

"It is *not* for you!" I hissed. "It is for *him*—for the Captain. And you *will* do it, or the boy remains as he is!"

He stood there in the pale light, with his mouth still open, and then he closed it softly, and nodded quietly, and brought me back to the jail.

29

The First Question

Third Week of September

"Problems!" boomed the Captain. "All kinds of problems! The minute you go back to your cell, all these problems come up, and I have to live with them for a whole week!"

I smiled. The great teachers—teachers like my Uncle back home, or Katrin—they love it when their students come back with problems about what they have taught them; it shows first of all that they were listening, and secondly that they are thinking. "Go ahead," I said. "Let's start with them. But one at a time please, and clearly stated."

He did that little frown of his and then went on, with an excitement that was lovely to see. "I mean, I've got lots of questions—but how about just one obvious one, first. I mean . . . " He paused, so he could say it right. "I mean, I had that bad back for years and years, before you fixed it, with the yoga . . . " And then suddenly he got stuck, even before he had reached where he'd gotten stuck.

"With the yoga?" it became a question now. "I mean, did you fix my back with the yoga, or did I just start *seeing* it different—as *fixed* rather than *hurt*—because, because, well—I guess because maybe the old seeds wore out, and some new seeds opened up?"

"It's a good question," I said first, "and one of the most important you could ask. And you have to buckle down and listen carefully if you really want to catch the answer." His little frown deepened into a positive scowl of concentration. I put my hand up to my face; middle finger between my eyebrows, thumb and pinky at the corners of my mouth, and pushed up. He gave a little laugh and loosened up his face, which had the effect of making his concentration even deeper.

"*How* your back got fixed was that you did the yoga. *Why the yoga worked* on you was that, yes, some different seeds in your mind began to assert themselves, and the old ones wore out."

"So what you're saying," he said, "is that—at some point in the past—I did something like, say, hit someone in the back." He gazed up at the ceiling, calculating, and then back down to me, with a tinge of embarrassment. "Or maybe, you could say, maybe I did it . . . did it a few times."

"Perhaps," I allowed.

"And then at some point the seeds I planted then—they ripen in my mind. And the images I had in my mind as I hurt someone's back, they come back in my mind, as my mind forces me to see my own back as hurting—the same way my mind makes me see the green stick as a pen, and the cow's mind makes her see it . . . "

"And *use* it," I added.

"See it, and *use* it," he continued, "as something good to eat."

"So far, so good," I said.

"And then after a while, those seeds—those *bad* seeds, I guess—they start to get old; they start to wear out . . . "

"As do *all things which do anything*," I added, "while they *do what they do*. The energy they have to do anything to us, or for us, wears out, simply *as they do it*." And I nodded at him to continue.

"And then, say, some other seeds that have been sleeping there in my mind, they wake up, and take over creating the images . . . "

"The *things*," I added.

"The images—the very things—that I see: in this case, the new seeds, they make me see . . . make me see my back as *cured*, as *fixed*."

"See, and *be*, fixed," I added.

He nodded. "And these new seeds, if there is any justice in the world—and you give me real hope now that there *is* real justice in the world—well, I suppose they must have been planted earlier on in my life: at some point when I did something . . . "

"And *watched* yourself do something," I added.

"Oh yes," he exclaimed. "Got to get that imprint into the mind, right. And so, these new seeds—must have been planted when I watched myself do something like, say, help a sick person—help someone in pain."

"Exactly," I said, again in admiration of his instincts.

"Which brings me to a *question*," he rattled on. "I mean, if it was the seeds in my own mind that made me see my back get better . . . "

"Made it *be* better," I added.

"Then why do yoga; why do yoga at all?" he beamed, with a glance to the center of the room. And it really was such a warm and muggy day that I couldn't blame him.

"Listen carefully," I said. "*The yoga made your back get better. It wouldn't* have made your back get better if you *hadn't* had seeds in your mind to *see* it get better. *The same seeds that made your back get better* made you *try* the yoga, made you attracted to it in the *first* place; *made* you think it might work; *made* me walk into your office that first day; *made* the Master's book be in my bag; *made* the poses and the sitting loosen the knot in the channels within your back. Do you see?"

He looked up at the ceiling for a quiet moment. It hadn't quite arrived, but he was close.

"But *if I had never tried the yoga,*" he pressed on, "those new seeds—the seeds to see myself get better—well they *still* would have opened up, and they *still* would have made me see my back get better."

"Not the point," I said softly. "Think hard. Think carefully. The fact is that they *did* open up, *when the yoga came to you,* and *when the yoga fixed you.* They made the yoga, *and* what the yoga did for you. You *had* to do the yoga, because you *did* do the yoga."

He looked at me steadily, really really trying hard to work it out. "It will come," I said. "And I'll tell you something. It helps a lot at this stage if you really ask all the Teachers, you see—your own Teacher, and your Teacher's Teacher, and so on all the way back to Master Patanjali and long long before him—ask them to help you. Ask them to come in their own invisible untouchable way and help you, help you to understand. And they will." I paused, so it would sink in. And then I said, "You haven't actually got to your first question, you know," I said with a smile.

"Oh yes . . . er . . . yes," he said, coming back to himself. He drew himself up like a real Captain then and proclaimed, "There's a problem with . . . with what you said . . . before, I mean." I smiled, wondering how many problems he'd find with the latest ideas.

"What I mean is," he went on, "is . . . well, let's say there really *is* some kind of justice—I mean, some kind of justice on a grand scale," and he waved his arms around big, to encompass not just the old mud jail but the entire universe just beyond its walls. "Well then—first of all—since my back hurt me for more than five years; and if, according to what you say, some kind of seeds in my mind made me see it that way all that time . . . "

"The way you see the pen," I nodded at the poor little stick, to remind him that we had both already agreed on this point.

"Well, yes—the way I see the pen—but anyway, that means that I must have beaten people on the back non-stop for five whole years, whereas . . . " he gazed up at the ceiling, calculating again " . . . whereas, I never did any such thing—I mean, never for any period of time even remotely . . . " He glared up and calculated again. The years with the Sergeant, cleaning up the gangs, I thought; they must have been something! "Even remotely," he repeated with confidence, "approaching five years in a row, so there seems to be a problem with this idea of seeds," he concluded.

"Ah," I said. "Seeds. We need to talk about seeds. We need to talk about how seeds work," I said.

"There is a short list of rules that governs how these seeds in our minds work; just as there are laws of nature that govern how, say, corn seeds work. We'll cover them today; it's not much, really.

"The Master opens this conversation with the first and most important rule of all. He says—

> *There is a connection*
> *Of cause and effect:*
> *The seeds ripen into*
> *Experiences refreshingly pleasant,*
> *Or painful in their torment;*

Depending on whether
You have done good to others,
Or done them wrong instead.

II.14

And so the first rule of the seeds—it's something you would guess, something you did guess, already—if there really is sort of a huge perfect justice in the world. And it's that—when you do any action at all that hurts someone—then a seed is planted in your mind which will ripen later on and make you see something unpleasant: cause you to have a painful experience. Equally so, whenever you do anything that helps someone, a seed is planted in your mind that will ripen and make you see something pleasant: an enjoyable experience. And remember that these seeds, again, are planted *simply by being aware* of yourself doing, saying, or even just thinking something which is positive or negative."

"That part's all right," he said, a little impatiently. "That's the whole attraction of this way of viewing the world: that bad things you do come back to you as pain, while good things come back to you as a pleasant experience, because of a sort of universal law that's as simple and airtight as say the law of gravity. And that thing about how *seeing* yourself do something presses the imprint into the mind—that's great. That goes a long way in making me believe the whole thing. But again: why *five entire years* of back pain, when I never did anything like that to anyone?"

"First things first," I cautioned him. "Now this first rule of how it all works says that nothing can ever happen otherwise: meaning, you can never expect a pleasant experience to develop from a negative action you've done, and never an unpleasant experience from a positive action you've done." I paused to let it sink in, and for everyone's automatic reaction to this idea to surface in his mind.

The Captain frowned a bit—didn't catch himself—and then blurted out, "Problem right there too—problem with the first rule, before you even got to my question. I mean, *what about all the things that people do that make other things happen at all*—and which obviously break this first rule of yours, right from the start?"

"Like what?" I challenged him.

The Captain glanced up at the ceiling. "Well, just about everything, really—it's so obvious. But all right, let's start with a simple one.

"You sit in your cell for three days and weave a nice Tibetan-style rug. The Sergeant takes it to town on market day, to one of the little trading stalls there. And he meets the owner and they begin to haggle over the price that the rug will fetch. At some point in the conversation, the Sergeant claims that the rug is worth double what he's been offered—and it doesn't matter *what* he's been offered, because he'll *always* say it's worth double that much—and he explains with a very straight face that it took his sister three *weeks* to weave this extraordinary *rug*, and there's *no way* he can take less money for it, or she and her child . . . I suppose that's the dog, you see . . . will surely die from hunger."

I smiled. "And so?"

"And so it works, you see: the lie works, and the man gives the Sergeant the full amount he was asking for. And there you have it: the very first rule of seeds is broken already. A *lie* produces a *wonderful profit*. And so it's not true that a negative action can only produce an unpleasant result.

"Unless you find extra money unpleasant," he mused quizzically, and shook his head. "No, no . . . can't say that the Sergeant would find extra money any problem at all."

But then he looked up at me, dead serious for the answer.

"It's *still* not your first question," I laughed; and he nodded, but we both knew it had to be answered.

"And so I give you the answer; the sacred answer to a question that has bothered all humankind for time with no beginning. How can an action which is clearly wrong have a desirable result? How can something like a shameless lie bring a person an extra profit?

"The answer is, you see, that the first rule *is not* broken. Extra money, for example, comes from an imprint *that was planted in the past* when the person involved—here, the Sergeant—was *generous* and *giving* to someone else. During the course of his discussion at the market, this seed *ripens,* and *forces* his mind to interpret some *heavy circular objects* as silver coins, being pressed into his hand by the person who has bought the rug.

"At the same time, the Sergeant has just pressed new imprints into his own mind, from his *negative act of lying* to someone else. At some point later on, these *new* seeds will ripen inside his own mind—and he will experience an *assortment of various sounds and tones* coming out of someone else's mouth as a pack of lies, meant to mislead *him.*

"What I mean to say, my dear Captain," and here I drew myself up very tall, the way that Katrin used to do at these same crossroads of elegant truth, "what I mean to say is, that *telling the lie had absolutely nothing to do with getting the extra money."*

The Captain just stared at me, and blinked only once over the next two minutes, passed in perfect silence. Then he stirred himself.

"But that's impossible, you see . . . ," he whispered. "Impossible—utterly impossible. Why, if what you just said is true, *then almost every single action undertaken by the millions upon millions of people in this entire world from hour to hour throughout their entire lifetimes doesn't at all bring them the things they thought those actions did.* It's impossible. Too much. How could . . . how could *everyone* . . . be so . . . so *wrong* . . . about . . . about *the most basic thing there is:* about how, why, anything we ever do ever works at all?"

"Perhaps," I answered softly, looking out the window. "Perhaps, somewhere in there, lies the clue . . . to why . . . all of us . . . end up . . . losing . . . everything, in the end."

And we never did reach his first question that day—but we did do the poses, and sitting down to give and take: planting the real causes.

30

The Gardening Begins

Fourth Week of September

"Forget those old problems!" exclaimed the Captain. "We have . . . why, we have tons of *new* ones!" But his face told me that they were only problems of clarification, and not of conviction. He had tasted a truly coherent idea of how our world actually works: an idea that made sense; an idea that showed there was a real justice behind things; and—most importantly—an idea that gave us, and all of those we love, everyone, a real way out of every kind of pain. And this knowledge had given his face a new glow, atop the healthy glow from the poses.

"I mean—first question. If the Sergeant *doesn't* lie about the rug, does he *still* get the extra money?"

"Of course," I said. "The lie and the extra money are in no way connected. There is no relationship of cause and effect between them *at all*. They just happen one right after the other, and so a part of our mind—a very wrong part of our mind—jumps on that and says, 'The lie brought the extra money. But the reason why a lie does not bring extra money is *so obvious that the entire population of our world for as long as our world has been around* has simply, terribly, overlooked it."

"What? How? How, if it is so obvious . . . how, by so many?"

"Seeds," I said bluntly. "But anyway, you must grasp this. Grasp this. If a lie was the real cause that brought you extra money, then every time you tried to get extra money by lying, *it should always work*. But it doesn't. It's that simple. It proves that the lie is not the real cause of the extra money."

He thought about it for a moment and that ancient powerful inner wind in the right-hand channel moved, as it had moved for time with no beginning, and it blinded him once more. But how much longer? We were shoving its energy into the middle channel, from the outside—and the inside.

For now though he missed the idea and spluttered, "But there are many other reasons why a lie might not always work to bring you extra money: someone else has told the person the truth; the person has found out you tend to lie; the person *doesn't care* if the weaver eats enough or not—anything."

"No," I said. "Think carefully; think bigger. Your very life depends upon it—and the lives of those two men out there, and . . . and the precious two you hope to find again. The *real cause of the extra money* should have—and did—actually *dictate* all the circumstances surrounding the entire event: the perceptions of the person who bought the rug; the perceptions of the Sergeant; the amount of money there; the fact that it was market day; the fact that the people and events all came together in exactly the way needed for the extra money to be paid: *this* is a *real* cause. *This* is what a *real* cause does.

"*A lie cannot cause extra money*. There is absolutely nothing similar between a lie and extra money. You may intentionally omitted.

as well expect a corn seed to grow into a watermelon. Lies *don't* work to get you extra money, because they *don't* make it come. You can lie, and maybe the money comes; or you can lie, and maybe it doesn't come. *Wake up, Captain! It's not the cause!"*

He sat back and breathed a giant sigh, then held his head with both hands, as if it were a balloon. "I mean," he said finally, "I mean it makes sense—it really does. But it's so . . . it's so . . . " He looked out the window. "It changes . . . so much . . . so much of what we do . . . so much of what we expect to work for us."

"And just think about this," I added. "What would happen, I mean . . . in the world . . . if, if everyone began to see what *really* causes things? What *really* causes extra money, for example?"

The Captain turned and looked out the window, and smiled ruefully. "Well, for one thing, if everyone realized that lying didn't—*couldn't*—ever work, well then, I suppose, we'd all just . . . just tell the truth, all the time."

I nodded, and let it sink in for a moment. "But to go back to your question—this last question, at least—yes, it's true. Even if the Sergeant hadn't lied, he would have gotten the extra money—because he already had the seeds for the extra money. I mean, someone who owed him an old forgotten debt would have showed up the same day, or perhaps an uncle somewhere would have left him some money in his will, something like that.

"And that leads us to some other rules about the seeds: that is, they cover *everything*, and they *never* go away, until they ripen."

"Cover everything,?" he said.

"Cover everything," I replied. "I mean, there's not *anything* around us or inside us which is *not* happening because of these seeds. *No good thing* can ever happen unless you have done something good to someone else, so that a seed can be planted and then ripen in your mind to make you see something as good. And *no bad thing* can ever happen unless you have done the opposite. Even the things that seem in-between, things that seem just neutral, neither good or bad, are happening because of background seeds planted by the very way we misunderstand our world just constantly.

"And from the other side, no seed is ever wasted: nothing we ever do, nothing we ever say, nothing we ever think ever *fails* to plant a seed. And each of these seeds will wait patiently in line, for years and years if necessary, to ripen upon us. They never, ever, 'forget.'

"And beyond that, there is one more important thing that you need to know about seeds: it is the answer to the first question you asked, before. Why did you have five years of back pain, if you never caused anyone else five years of any similar pain?"

I opened my hand, and pushed a pit from a mango fruit into his palm. It was from the first fruit I'd ever gotten in my cell, a few days before. You see, towards the end of the season, there is no food in India *cheaper* than a mango. They all fall down at nearly the same time.

"How much does it weigh?" I asked.

He lifted the pit in his hand. "A few ounces," he replied, "can't be more than that."

And then I pulled him to the window, to look at the struggling little mango tree outside.

"And that tree—if it ever gets watered and tended properly—how much will it weigh?"

"Why I don't know," he said. "I suppose, in time, a few thousand pounds at least."

"Right," I said, and we sat down again. "And so it's something—something very important, that you must understand. Seeds . . . seeds in the mind, over time, they grow: they expand, and get bigger, just as much as seeds in nature do. And they *never* get old waiting to ripen; they *never* just go away. There is nothing in the mind to make them age or spoil the way that physical seeds do. And so, you see, even just hitting another person on the back once— for a few minutes—it could easily cause you five years of pain in your back, later."

The Captain suddenly choked, and then stared down at the ground, and then looked up again at me, almost angrily.

"Impossible!" he spluttered. "Impossible!"

"What impossible?" I replied calmly.

"Out of the question!" he exclaimed. "Five years of pain, for a few moments of . . . of excess . . . in the heat of anger? What kind of justice is that? I thought there was some kind . . . some kind of *justice* here! Why . . . why that would make the result of the seed, well, I don't know . . . something like . . . something like thousands of times greater than the seed itself . . . "

And he faltered then and we both gazed down again at the mango pit, still lying in my palm.

"No! Too much!" he exclaimed again. "I can't believe that a seed in the mind would grow like those outside seeds do—I mean, thousands of times bigger than when they were planted."

I waved around at the room. "Who does this room belong to?" I asked.

"Why, to the King," he replied. "Ultimately, it belongs to the King, the King of the Realm."

"And how long . . . how long has the Realm existed?" I asked. I had no idea, and it didn't matter anyway. All countries start out basically the same way.

"Why, this is now the 14th Dynasty!" said the Captain proudly. "Over six centuries, since the Great Council."

"Great Council?" I asked.

"Why, yes," he said, shocked that I had missed out on the entire history of another of our planet's momentary empires. "That is where they drew up . . . the Great Law."

"Great Law?" I asked.

Now the Captain looked positively scandalized at my ignorance. "The Great Law, of course," he insisted. "Setting forth the structure of the Realm—a whole new idea in government."

"Idea?" I asked. "Whose idea?"

"Why, as everyone knows—or should know—the vision of the Great Forefather, for a new and better country."

I paused for a moment. "Started out as an idea in someone's mind then." His eyes narrowed.

"And how many stations are there like this one—a hundred? Several hundred? And thousands of other buildings, with tens of thousand of people working, to govern—how many—hundreds of thousands more? Has not one idea, in one man's mind, has it not grown into this, this country, and the idea of it, in thousands and thousands of minds? Do not ideas begin and grow and then spread, fantastically, just like any other seeds? Are not even the hopes that drive people to work at an occupation for their entire lifetimes, for decades, born in a single idea as they begin their careers? Come on, Captain. Mental seeds don't grow any less than mango pits, and probably a lot more."

He looked stunned—as anyone who really grasped what we had just said should have been—and he began a few minutes' silent review of his entire life, I think. And then he said, as anyone at this point should say too, "But . . . but is there anything we can do? I mean . . . I mean, there are so many . . . so many things, so many mistakes in every person's life. Can these seeds . . . can they be changed, before they ripen? Is there anything like a counter-seed? Or any special way of creating very powerful *good* seeds?"

"Oh Captain," I said. "It is the perfect question. And the answer is yes; of course yes, or it would all be so impossible. We have a job—we all have a job to do. We have to try to get at the old bad seeds—the ones already planted in our minds in the past, by mistake. Whatever old good seeds we have need reinforcement, and cultivating. From now on, we need to be careful only to plant good new seeds, and never negative ones.

"We need to learn every detail about how the seeds operate, and how to create some new super-seeds that would be powerful enough even to change the way we see the mortal nature of our bodies, and more. In short, we must become experts at the intelligent management of our mental seeds. As the Master puts it in his *Short Book*,

> *We must become*
> *As gardeners.*
>
> IV.3B"

The Captain nodded resolutely, still obviously shaken by the review of the seeds he knew he possessed already. We went through the poses, and the silent wishes for his men. And at the end of the sitting he opened his eyes and said to me, "The strangest thing has happened."

"What's that?"

"Ravi—I mean, the Sergeant—he has asked me, he has asked me . . . to give him some lessons, in yoga!"

I tried to look sufficiently surprised, but the Captain wasn't really paying any attention to me anyway. Instead, his eyes were wide open, unseeing, in some kind of minor panic.

"Well, what do you think I should do?" he said.

"Do?" I asked. "Why, why teach him, of course . . . help him, to the best of your ability."

"But I . . . but I, I've never done anything like that before, you know. I'm . . . I'm not even quite sure . . . where to start."

"That's the easy part," I assured him. "Get him . . . get him to do his yoga for someone else's sake—to help someone else. You can't go wrong from there. Best kind of seed there is."

The Captain nodded gratefully. "Makes sense," he said, and then paused, with a mixture of emotions passing across his face. "And . . . ," he continued then.

"Yes?"

"And . . . he has asked, he asks if he may bring his son . . . here, to the jail . . . to have classes . . . classes with you."

"I love to teach children," I said. "They are wonderful students. Very open-minded to new ideas, even very big ones."

"But that's not . . . ," he stumbled. "It's not . . . that, you see . . . it's that, well, he . . . he has a fairly serious . . . serious problem, you see—he was hurt; he was . . . burned, you see, rather seriously . . . in an accident." The Captain paused again. "Frankly, I'm not sure you'll be able to help him."

I looked at the Captain steadily, and Katrin came in to me again—it felt so wonderful, whenever that happened. "Captain," I said, "there's one thing you must be very clear about."

"What's that?" he said.

"It's about *things*," I said. "The way we make *things*: the way our mind makes us see things—the way that things, all things, really happen. You see, if the way something like a pen really happens is that seeds in our own minds are forcing

213

us to see it that way; and if we can change seeds like this around with some kind of seed management—with what the Master calls 'gardening'; then it doesn't really matter how *big* a thing is, you see? I mean, the same rules apply to pens, and to sore backs, and to bodies that die, and to loved ones that have left us, and to terrible injuries, and to . . . " I waved my arms around us " . . . and to *whole worlds*."

31

Breaking the Circle

When the boy arrived, he absolutely refused to come inside the bars. The Sergeant did everything a good father would do—from playfulness to sternness—but nothing worked.

Finally I said, "Sergeant, sir, just leave him out there on the bench, with something to play with. And then, if you would, please, just leave my door open, and . . . please, I think it will help . . . if you could bring my little dog in . . . "

His face darkened ever so slightly, but his new leaf was still turned over, and he grudgingly brought me Long-Life. We had a wonderful play together — it was the first time he'd seen my cell from the inside. We were both resting it off, out of breath, in the front corner when the boy wandered over—very cautiously—and gave my little lion that look that says, "Can I pet you too?" And of course he could, and the boy was inside before he knew it.

"Now my puppy, you see," I said first, "he's been all tied up out back for the longest time. And so his legs, you see," I held him up between us, "have got all short, you see."

215

The boy nodded in sympathy. "And so, it would really be a big help to him, and to *me*, you see, because we often have to walk long ways together, if you . . . if you could, you see, come in before class a little early each time, and give him a good pet all over, but especially on his *legs*, you see."

And the boy nodded, quietly, and we started some new seeds going there, in the garden of his mind. Before he left, he told me his name was Ajit: the Undefeatable, and truly his heart was so.

φ

"The most important principle a mental-seed gardener needs to know is called The Circle," I said next to the Captain.

"Circle?" he queried.

"Circle," I repeated. "You see, the way bad seeds work is very, very nasty. The worst thing about bad seeds it that they make us plant *more* bad seeds. Sort of how all the crops that ever were in the world were only able to happen because there were seeds saved over from the crops of the year before . . . get the idea?" The Captain nodded.

"Now the Master is talking about this idea when he says,

> *And these negative thoughts*
> *Are their very root.*
>
> II.12A"

"Which negative thoughts?" asked the Captain. "And whose root?"

"We spoke about them already," I said, "but this is where we tie it all together, because you need this to do the gardening well.

"Let's choose a real example, and then I can show you how The Circle works. Let's pretend say that you have a boss, here in the station. And let's say that—like a lot of bosses—he walks in every once in a while and screams at you, usually for something you didn't do anyway."

"Not difficult to imagine," replied the Captain, obviously recalling his old days in the capital.

"Now the first step in The Circle is that habit we are born with: the one the Master was talking about when he said, 'We misunderstand our world: things that are not themselves seem to us as if they were.' He means, for example, that we are *born* with the habit of believing that a pen is a pen by itself, and not because seeds are going off in our mind and making us see it as a pen. And the *proof* that it's not a pen by itself is . . . "

"The cow thing; I remember," he said, a little petulantly, but it was important to remind him that we were already all agreed on that part.

"Step two in The Circle is what the Master called 'selfness,' meaning the tendency to believe that things are happening by themselves, from *their* side, as it awakens again in us even in the womb, triggered by our first experiences of other objects."

"I recall that . . . pretty well," remarked the Captain, but I saw from his eyes that he was still with me.

"Step three," I continued. "A specific object, like your yelling boss—something that makes you feel strongly, either good or bad—steps into your day. The tendency to believe that *he is bad by himself*, that he is *bad from his own side*, suddenly comes upon you so strong that your misunderstanding graduates into what the Master called 'grasping.'

"And maybe, remember, maybe you've already learned the thing about the pen—I mean, maybe you *already understand* that your screaming boss is just like the pen: that *you* are experiencing an unpleasant boss at that moment only because *certain seeds* are going off in your own mind, forcing you to see what is otherwise just an odd collection of colors and shapes and sounds as a boss who is screaming at you. And of course he's not unpleasant *by himself*, from *his own side*, even in that tense moment, because . . . " I paused to let him fill it in.

"Because, well, I guess . . . " he needed only a second to think about it " . . . because, you see, there could be another office worker sitting right next to you—say, a rival for the position the boss himself gave you a few months before—and this other worker will probably perceive this *same boss*, at this *same difficult moment*, as someone quite reasonable, who has finally become aware of how truly incompetent *you* are."

"Just so," I said. "And you see, a boss who is unpleasant *by himself*, a boss who is unpleasant *from his own side*, could never also be *reasonable* or *pleasant* at the very same moment, could he? No more than a pen that could simultaneously be a confection, you see?"

"So far, so good," smiled the Captain.

"Good," I repeated. "So at step three we already have you *grasping* onto the screaming boss as something unpleasant—from his own side, and not because there are unpleasant *seeds* ripening within your *own* mind and making you see him that way.

"And by the way," I sped it past him, "what kind of negative action do you think you'd have to have done in the past to get this unpleasant boss yelling at you now?"

"Oh, I don't know," he said off-handedly. "I guess you must have yelled like that at someone *else*, before."

"Right," I said, and rolled ahead. "So on to step four in The Circle: having forgotten now that what you are seeing—and *hearing*—in front of you is happening because of seeds *which you planted yourself,* you begin to *dislike* the boss. You get angry at him. Something akin to blaming your toe because you stubbed it.

"And this chain of negative thoughts, you see—seeing things wrong as this habit came into life with you; seeing things wrong even as you see your first things; *grasping* to this wrong way of seeing things under pressure; and then finally *disliking* something, strongly, because of your misunderstanding—they are what the Master calls the *very root* of the other two."

"What other two?" asked the Captain.

"You tell me," I said. "What happens when your dislike for the yelling boss—however misinformed it may be—gets strong enough?"

"Well, that's easy," answered the Captain, his eyes misting over as he recalled his big-office days. "You yell *back* at him!"

"Right," I said. "And so this chain of negative thoughts has triggered what the Master called 'the things we do': step number five in The Circle. And the things we do, they 'plant the storehouse,' as he said it. Which is step number six: we plant new seeds in our minds."

"Seeds to see," he said, the whole process suddenly dawning on him, "seeds to see . . . another . . . person . . . yelling at us, in the future." He paused.

"Oh my goodness," he said, clutching his head in that way he'd developed ever since we'd started talking about the seeds. "Oh my goodness. What you're saying is that . . . is that our most *natural* and *automatic* response to the negative things that happen to us all day is . . . is precisely the *one and only* action that would plant the seeds for us to see *the very same thing* happening to us again. It's all . . . one . . . huge . . . vicious . . ."

"*Circle*," I said. And I smiled, despite the vicious circle. Because the first thing you need to stop an enemy is to know *who he is*, and the Captain had just gotten over that hurdle.

"And you need to see," I went on, "you need to see one more thing: how this all ties back into the channels, and the subtle winds that flow within them; what we talked about from the very beginning, with your bad back." His hand went again, automatically, from his head to where he used to hold his back.

"We spoke about two main *bad* channels, that twist around the middle channel, and choke it at certain points . . . "
"The channels called 'sun' and 'moon,' running down close on either side of the spine," he recalled.

"Right," I said. "And if you also remember, we said that within them run two very basic, negative types of inner wind—tied to the two most basic, negative thoughts."

"I remember," he said, chewing on his lip with concentration. "Mistaken thoughts about *things* running on the right, in the sun channel; and mistaken thoughts about our own thoughts, and our own mind—about what we use to *see* things—running on the left, in the moon channel."

"Exactly," I said. "And now you can begin to appreciate just what a problem these two channels and their two inner winds are . . . "

"Well, the thoughts that ride upon their winds—according to what we've been talking about these last few days—are the very root of all our trouble; I mean, that most basic tendency, born inside us as we ourselves are born, to misunderstand ourselves and everything around us."

"Right again," I said, and then I paused for a moment, looking out the window. "I mean," I said, "if you were really tired of having bosses—or anyone else—scream at you, what is the one thing you'd want to avoid at all costs?"

"Screaming at others," he said simply, truly.

"But what if the boss screaming at you makes you very upset, and you are just about to scream back?"

"Well, I guess you'd have to stop, and catch yourself—even though it might be very difficult in the heat of the moment. You'd have to stop, and say to yourself. 'Whoa now! Wait just a minute. I have to see this boss screaming at me now because of seeds I put in my own mind in the past, when I screamed at someone else. No way I'm going to set that vicious cycle in motion one more time!' And then, I think, if you tried to remember this—no matter how much he screamed, no matter how upset you felt—then you'd have a good chance of breaking the cycle, The Circle, right where it starts."

"Perfect," I smiled. "And if you were able, in that one most difficult moment, to keep all this in mind—then *which channel do you think your thoughts would be running in?*"

He paused, and then answered, "Well, since it's such a *right* thought, then I guess it would have to be cracking into the middle channel, at least a little."

"Just so," I said. "And any small amount of wind moving in the middle channel also means that much *less* wind to move in the side channels."

"And so it would loosen up knots *all over your body,*" he mused. "The most powerful bad winds, getting deflated. You'd feel happier, and . . . and your body, well, it would just naturally get more and more healthy and strong." Then he stopped, abruptly.

"Miss Friday, *what would happen if you could get all the winds into the middle channel?*"

I smiled on the outside and sang on the inside. He was getting close. But all I said was, "It's coming," the way Katrin would have.

"What I really wanted to point out now," I continued, "is just that it's hard to remember all this at that one crucial moment when you most need to: when the boss is actually in your face, screaming. And so you'd want to give yourself the best chance you could, to remember. I mean, you'd want to *practice* thinking about how it's really your own mind that makes you see things; you'd want to stop at odd moments throughout your day and practice just *thinking this way* for a minute or two.

"That in itself would head some of the inner winds towards the middle channel, giving the side channels less power every minute you could keep this kind of thinking up. Spending as well a few minutes now and then to practice taking away others' troubles, and giving them what they wish for—even just mentally—would have the same effect.

"And there is, of course, one last very *practical, doable* way of heading inner winds towards the middle channel. It's going at it the other way around: instead of working on your thoughts, which are like horsemen atop the horses, you go and work directly on the inner winds. It's like coming and taking the reins of a horse and walking him down a different road—and then the person riding on his back comes along automatically. We move the *winds* on purpose, and then the *thoughts* riding atop them are forced to come along . . . "

"Why, you do *yoga*," exclaimed the Captain, catching on. "You do the yoga poses—the exercises. Because if you do them right, they loosen up the knots almost by brute force: knocking on the pipes. And then at least some small amount of wind is sent towards the middle channel, by definition, as the knots are relaxed. And because some number of your thoughts are riding on these winds, some number of your thoughts themselves are already directed to the middle channel. And thoughts that start going . . . to the middle channel . . . are changed, are they?"

"They are," I nodded.

"Doing the yoga . . . doing the yoga exercises," he said excitedly. "It . . . then it actually *gets you ready to have the ideas we've been talking about.* You hear them, and then you *grasp* them . . . better . . . if you've already been doing the *poses,*" he raced on. "Why, it's probably even why . . . "

"Why you yourself have been able to get all this stuff," I said with a smile. "And even why you just got *why* you get this stuff," I beamed. "Sort of like, you see, starting a *good* version of The Circle, building up its own power to keep itself going."

"Poses help winds help thoughts help poses again; why, I never would have thought of that!" he fairly squealed. And then I took him through a really hard yoga session, so he wouldn't forget how good it was for him and his winds.

32

The Fortress
of Little Things

Second Week of October

The corporal led me back to my cell that day, and we ran into the Sergeant standing in front of Busuku's cell, screaming and banging his stick on the bars.

"Idiot!" he blustered, "Why . . . why, you can't even steal a cow right! So what makes you think you could get *this* right?"

"Idiot, am I?" roared Busuku, nose-to-nose with the Sergeant through the bars, his chubby face red and his little belly quaking. "Well just come inside here for one minute, you brainless thug, without that stick, and I'll *show* you!"

"Show me what?" raved the Sergeant.

"The *Knuckle Pose*," bellowed Busuku. And then he caught sight of the corporal and me and screamed out, "Miss Friday! Miss Friday! Come over here for a moment, if you please." And then, to the Sergeant, "We can settle this right here and now, you know."

The corporal ambled over to the two still clutching my arm, his mouth wide open at all the excitement.

"Good," exclaimed Busuku, his jowls shaking. "Now Miss Friday, listen to this. The Sergeant here, after three or four whole lessons with the Captain, you see, he says he's learned the *right* way of doing the Mountain Pose from him, and he says the way *I* do it is all wrong."

I smiled and started to answer, but the Sergeant butted in. "I didn't say that the *Captain* taught me the *right* way, you *idiot*; I said I *figured out the best way* to do the Mountain Pose."

"On your *back*, you said!" Busuku looked at me with the eyes of a condemned prisoner, pleading for his life. "Please . . . please . . . Miss Friday. I mean, *can you believe it? I* mean, the very first pose of all, the pose where—where *any* fool at all would know—you are just *standing* there, getting ready, getting ready to start something like Bowing to the Sun! And this . . . this . . . miserable . . . excuse . . . for an Officer of the Law, he says, you start it on your back! *Can you believe it?* Tell him! Tell him it ain't so!"

I opened my mouth again, but again the Sergeant cut me off. "Look, Busuku. If you had any brains, you'd just get down and *do* it the way I said. And then if it's wrong, well Miss Friday—and even the corporal; I mean, *anybody—*could see it was wrong, in a second."

"Well that's just what I'll do, then!" cried Busuku, and he flopped down on the floor, on his back, with his mighty belly pointing to the sky.

There was a moment of silence.

"Like I said," declared the Sergeant. "There it is: the *Mountain* Pose." And without another word he turned and walked back to the room in the front.

Busuku laid on the floor, staring in rage at the ceiling. The corporal was silent for a full two minutes, and then turned to me with a look of surprise.

"I think," he said then, "I *think*, that . . . that the Sergeant . . . he . . . he has . . . made . . . a *joke*!" And he stood there in shock, as did I and . . . and poor Busuku as well.

φ

At our next class I came into the Captain and said, "Time to get down to some basic gardening. I mean, the Master at this point jumps straight into explaining what the most powerful good seeds to plant are. It's a short list, and it's designed to save us all time, by getting us right into the most crucial kinds of seeds we should be planting. And the Master presents them in such a way that we also learn their opposites: the kinds of actions that plant really bad seeds— the actions we want to avoid. And then along the way, as we work through the list, I thought we could keep going over more of the questions that will naturally come up in your mind about how the seeds work to produce our world."

"You're the teacher!" exclaimed the Captain, and I knew immediately that he had begun to experience the difficulty of it himself. Sort of a sweet revenge that teachers get when their students take on pupils of their own.

"Thank you!" I said sunnily. "Now the Master gives the first powerful way of planting new good seeds when he says,

> *The first form of self-control*
> *Is avoiding harm to anyone.*
> II.30A

The 'self-control' part is obvious . . . ," I began.

"Seems like the whole key is self-control," said the Captain. "I mean, trying to control our old instincts, because they just keep us going around and around in that Circle of trouble: bad seeds from yelling at someone before make us see the boss yelling at us now; and then our natural instinct is to yell back; which happens to be the best way . . . "

"The *only* way!" I exclaimed.

"The exact, best, and *only* way to plant *more* seeds to see *more* bosses yelling at us in the future." But then he hesitated, and frowned a bit.

"Little problem with that," he said. "Okay if I ask?"

It was good that he was careful about not interrupting the flow of the class; but this was a great way to flow, if I guessed correctly what he was about to ask. "Go ahead," I said.

"Well suppose that someone does come in and starts yelling, at you or someone; what are you *supposed* to do? I mean, just let them go on, realizing that it's your own seeds? And what if say they go even further, and start hitting someone?" he asked.

"Beautiful, beautiful question," I replied. "And the answer is that *we have to act*. We have to try our very best to stop violence done to anyone; and by doing so we plant lots of *good* seeds, you see. But as we try to prevent violence being done, we can *never* do so with hatred or anger, you see—because *that* would be planting very powerful *bad* seeds. We must try to restrain others who do violence, without violence—especially without thoughts of violence.

"And I'll ask you another question," I said, "and it's a little difficult. You have to think clearly." His face got that look of official duty, but he was careful not to do his concentration scowl.

"Suppose we do come across someone yelling at someone else, or even trying to hurt them physically. And suppose we try to restrain them—without malice, and without violence. Suppose further that we *succeed* in doing so, and they stop hurting the other person. I ask you; why has the violence stopped?"

The Captain nodded, and then *did* scowl with concentration, and finally looked back into my eyes. "Why . . ." he said, in some wonder, "why, I suppose that— the violence has stopped, *for the person to whom it was being committed*—because . . . because *their own seeds*, planted *in their own minds*, by *themselves*, in the past, have . . . well, they've *changed*. The bad seeds, I suppose, have flowered and spent whatever power they had, and disappeared. And now new seeds have ripened to take their place in the flow of the person's day—in the flow of their very life—and these new seeds are forcing them to see the violence *stop*."

He paused then, before that crucial hurdle in thinking that we must all one day leap over, and leave forever behind us.

"But then . . . but then, *it doesn't really matter* whether I try to help or not," he said, almost painfully. "If the person being hurt has seeds to see my efforts *help* them, then they will. If they don't have any seeds like that, then my efforts *won't* help them. So why make the efforts at all?"

I nodded. "This is one of the most important questions of all, and you have to listen carefully to the answer, and never forget it. Otherwise you could one day fall off what great Masters of the past have called the 'Cliff of the Great Mistake.'

"There are several issues here. First of all, if you notice, we have just explained precisely why it *doesn't always work* when you try to help someone else, no matter how hard you try, or how good your intentions are. That in itself is a sacred lesson, and will prevent you from ever becoming bitter or hesitant to continue helping others, should one or two such efforts fail to work out. It will give you the strength and the clarity to know that, regardless, you *must* continue to help others—you *must* devote your life to it.

"Secondly, it's important to realize that the person you may be helping the most is the *person who was committing the violence* . . . " I paused to let him pick up the thread of the thought.

"Because . . . well, because—he is in the process of planting tremendous negative seeds in his own mind: he is inflicting future pain *upon himself* which far exceeds whatever he is doing to his victim at the moment." And then the Captain added, "Because of the way that seeds grow into things so much bigger than themselves."

"Exactly," I said. "So really your act of kindness here is towards the person *doing* the violence. That's why it's so crucial that you avoid *hating* him as you try to restrain him."

"You stop him . . . because you *love* him," murmured the Captain. Such sweet thoughts.

"And then finally," I said, "you are doing sort of a cosmic public service whenever you risk yourself to stand up against violence. First of all, people see your example; they take hope, and they follow it. Secondly—and here's perhaps the *kindest* thing you are doing—you are consciously planting extraordinary new seeds in your *own* mind when you take a stand against violence being done to another. If you truly master this ultimate form of gardening—if you succeed in working with your own seeds so well that the inner channels undergo a profound change, and you become a being of pure light within a world of the same light—well then you really have a gift to offer to all of livingkind, and you will."

"Because whatever you have done yourself, you can show others how to do too," mused the Captain. "I see, Miss Friday. I see; I really see. And thank you for that."

We paused both of us for a moment, both dreaming of that day. And then I took us back to the Master's first form of self-control.

"So self-control," I said, "as the Master means it—it's just keeping yourself from making problems for yourself, for the you you will be later on down the road. It's really just being nice to a you that you haven't *been* yet, you see?" The Captain nodded.

"And that's one of the most important ideas in the Master's whole book, you see," I said from my heart. "It's the whole thing about working with seeds—with gardening. We are really just trying to shape our future; and it's exciting, you see, because since everything works through seeds then we finally have a choice in the matter: we can consciously and purposely design and build our own future into a garden paradise. We are finally in control of what happens in our lives; or rather, we are in control of what *will happen* in our lives. As the Master puts it,

> *The pain that we*
> *Are ridding ourselves of*
> *Is all the pain*
> *That would have come to us*
> *In the future.*
>
> II.16

It means, you can't stop the pain of the present moment, just by wishing it, or working at it in ways that life has already shown us don't really work. You can't put your hand on a huge mango tree and push it back into the ground—it's too late. We have to deal at the level of seeds—of seeds *before* they start growing into the huge things they will become. We are gardening . . . for the future."

"But how long?" demanded the Captain. "How far into the future? How long does it take before the seeds we are working with today give their effect, in the future?"

"It's coming," I said. "We'll get to that—we have to get to it. But I can tell you now that there are ways—special ways—of making the seeds grow almost instantaneously. And of course I will teach them to you; I must.

"Now back to the idea of self-control; of learning not to lay things around your cosmic house that you're just going to stub your own toe on later. And that's all the point I was trying to make; I know that the word 'self-control' smacks of rules, and punishment, and guilt—and I want to make very sure that you never think of it that way here in the Master's *Short Book.* Self-control here is simply the *art of avoiding future pain for yourself:* avoiding new bad seeds in your own mind."

"*That* kind of self-control sounds more like . . . like a pleasure," replied the Captain.

"Good," I said. "And now we should get on to what it means to 'avoid harming anyone.' The Master here is beginning a discussion of things we do physically, with our bodies, which plant powerful seeds. Later on he'll get into things we do with our words—with what we say—and then lastly things we do just by thinking. And so here he's saying, at the very beginning, that we can plant immense good seeds if we are careful never to cause anyone physical harm."

"It makes a lot of sense that he starts with that," the Captain thought out loud. "If our whole goal with yoga is to clear up problems with our health—to make our bodies and our hearts strong and clear—then of course the seeds we'd want to avoid the most are those that deal with harming others."

I looked out the window for a moment, and then came back to him. "That last thing you said—about 'harming others'—it gives me a thought. I mean, you know what it is to hurt someone physically; we don't need to talk about that. So perhaps the most important thing we could do today is to talk about some grey areas—some ways of causing harm that are not so obvious—and also talk a bit about the practical details.

"By 'practical details,' I mean that—well, suppose you go up to someone and tell them that avoiding physical harm to others is the key to success in yoga: that if you have in your mind seeds of never hurting others, then you will get very good at the poses and the sitting and breathing, and it will all have an extraordinary effect on your body, and your happiness too. The normal reaction you get from most people though is something like, 'Well, actually, I don't have any problems that way at all. I have never say killed or seriously injured a person, and almost never in my life struck another person. So I would guess that yoga should start working well for me right away.' But then maybe it only works for them some, or only slowly, or maybe not much at all.

"And they start to wonder why, and it's important right then to explain these seeds to them carefully, so they can do something about it right away, and start getting real results before they get discouraged.

"You see, the vast majority of the seeds that run our lives haven't come from major events like murdering another person, or stealing all the money say from the business we work for. It's not large single actions that plant most of our seeds; rather, it's the small actions, and words, and thoughts, that we do on a constant basis over the length of a lifetime.

"And so when we want to turn the seeds around, the best way is to start with the very small, continual things we do from day to day. If we're trying to learn not to harm others, for example, we might just look around us for small ways that we can protect the health and lives of others. Maybe it's just picking a piece of paper up off the floor, because someone might come along and slip on it, and hurt themselves. Maybe it's just deciding not to talk or eat while we drive a cart down the road, knowing that one day the distraction could cause us to hurt someone seriously, by accident. Maybe it's going out of our way to say something encouraging to someone at work who seems tense, knowing that this emotion will hurt them physically if they keep it up over a few years' time.

"What I'm talking about is maintaining a constant, modest, joyful state of mind which is always looking for ways to protect others from harm—all day long, just in the little world we live in. This is the most powerful and at the same time most enjoyable way to plant the seeds in our mind that would take us to the highest goals of life."

The Captain started looking around at the papers that still covered a good part of the floor of his office. It was a good start.

"Concentrating on the small things has another advantage," I said. "We call it the Fortress Principle. If you're a great king with lots of treasure and family to protect, you might want to build a wall around your palace. And then just to make sure that no one ever breaches that wall you might want to put in a moat around the outside of the wall: nobody gets over the wall, because they never even get past the moat. And then if you're really serious you might plant a lot of nasty thorn bushes all around the outside of the moat itself: because if no one ever even gets as far as the moat, then certainly no one will ever get through the wall.

"So it's like a group of concentric circles: rings of protection within rings of protection. Having an enemy break through the outside ring represents, say, causing harm to anyone else even by accident, or negligence. If you are always careful and aware not to harm others this way, then you will obviously never do someone a *small* harm on purpose, which would be like having the enemy slip across the moat.

"And if you never purposely do a *small* harm to someone, then of course you will never see your enemy break through the inside wall, which would be something very serious: say, killing another human being intentionally. And so living with the small things; thinking constantly, all day, about even very small things we can do to protect the lives and happiness of others—simple, powerful, *consideration* for those around us, really—is the key to the treasure house of the seeds within our minds."

I looked up at the Captain and decided he needed a break; it was a lot to digest in one day. "I'll tell you what," I said. "You try over the next week to think about some of those grey areas—about things that may or may not cause harm to others: things you're not quite sure about. Have them ready when we start, next time."

The Captain smiled; he loved questions, and that's what made him such a perfect student. Of course I was still careful not to tell him so, because you know a big head *doesn't* make a perfect student, or teacher.

33

Difficult Questions and Difficult Answers

Third Week of October

For a lone prisoner inside a mud jail out in the middle of nowhere, my schedule was beginning to get oddly packed. There were the classes with the Captain; and the rugs to weave; and the increasingly less secret sessions with Busuku at night through the wall (I was never *totally* sure he was doing things right, but he certainly grunted in the right places); and of course the lessons with the Sergeant's boy, Ajit. He had very powerful seeds within him from the start, and it was more simply a task of awakening them. His leg was already improving, and I was always watching for ways of getting at his seeds from the inside. What he needed most was to be around more people, so he'd have more people to help and serve.

One day just after dusk the corporal came out of the side room for perhaps the tenth time, looking oddly out the door to the road, and then back at my cell. I thought he might be expecting someone, but so far I had only seen one person ever come to visit him: the woman who brought a large jug of water to the jail twice a day. The water was drawn

235

from a public well down the road towards town; every jug meant standing in line for at least an hour. Not that anyone minded; this was where people had a chance to see each other, and talk, and find out the town gossip. And then the lady would come with the jug and put it on the porch, and sometimes the Sergeant or even the Captain would come out for the latest news, and exchange the usual banter that working men and a lady who comes like that so often do.

And so finally the corporal walks stiffly to the door of my cell; but first he turns to Busuku's and says, "Mr. Busuku, I . . . I need to ask you a favor, if you will."

"What's that, my young fellow?" he answers lazily.

"Well . . . you see . . . I, I—tonight, I mean, right now, in fact—I am . . . I am going to take Miss Friday . . . take her . . . somewhere . . ."

I hear Busuku getting up off the floor in a (comparative) flash, ready to defend my honor again.

"Young man!" he says.

"Oh . . . it's nothing, sir . . . you see, what I want to do . . . is . . . is take her home, to see my mother, you see. To see if . . . if she can help her, the way she is helping everyone else, you see, sir."

"Ah," says Busuku, knowingly. "Well that . . . I think that would be wonderful."

"And one thing, sir, you see—it would be, you know, a real help to me if . . . if, you see, the Sergeant and the Captain . . . "

"My lips are sealed," says Busuku, with a little chuckle. "But don't dawdle, my boy . . . "

"Oh yes; the Sergeant," squeaks the corporal.

"Sergeant, my arse," growls Busuku. "I just don't want to miss my secret class tonight with Miss Friday, son. So make sure she's home on time."

"Yes sir," replies the corporal, his voice quivering. And then the crossbar is up off the door, and he is leading me down the road in the growing dark.

We walked a long distance, out in the opposite direction from town. The corporal kept his head down and we stepped off the road whenever anyone came the other way. Then at some point he turned onto a side road that meandered off to the left through a silent forest of tall, single trees growing far apart from each other. It was all completely silent.

And then we came to a clearing, and a simple but pretty and well-kept cottage of thatched reeds. Inside there was a wide, clean room with a well-worn, spotless floor of packed clay. In the middle of the room was a mat of woven rushes, and upon it a small, low round wooden table with a lamp made of a wick and melted butter in a lovely little clay dish. And in the halo of golden light there was a woman, an old woman, sitting soft and quiet, wrapped in an elegantly simple white cotton *sari* dress. She greeted me with bright, loving eyes beneath calm—almost sleepy—eyelids.

"My mother," said the corporal in introduction. "Miss Friday," he said to Mother. And then he stooped shyly at a water jug and poured us each a cup of clean, cool water.

"You may call me Mata Ji," she said, and I smiled. It meant "Mother," in any language. And then she reached to hand me one of the cups, but she could only push it to me slowly, across the top of the table. And I saw that her hands were bent and twisted: the backs curved backwards, the wrong way, and the fingers locked straight away from them.

The corporal cleared his throat, and said nervously, "You see, Mata Ji has . . . has this problem . . . with . . . with her hands . . . " Then he looked to her for help, as I suppose he often did.

"My son Chandra has told me a lot about you," continued the woman gracefully. And then abruptly she simply grasped my hands clumsily but warmly between her own, and closed her eyes. And we were silent like that for—I don't know how long. Everything just felt wonderful, and silent, and very very peaceful.

And then she opened her eyes again and a small tear made its way down her cheek, and she turned to her son and said, "It will work, Chandra; she is as you said she was. Very much like a woman who came into our lives long ago, in the year you were born. Yes, very much like . . . like *her*," she smiled, gazing into my face.

"Will you . . . please . . . be so kind, as to teach me yoga? Repair what age has done to me?" she asked, in a warm wave of humility.

"Of course, but of course," was all I could say, and held the incredible warmth of her hands in mine. And then I gazed at the corporal's face, so full of hope and joy, but so tormented by his dullness—and I added, "But there is one condition. Your son . . . your son must agree to begin lessons in yoga too, from . . . from the Captain."

The woman arched an eyebrow in surprise, and looked to the corporal. "Chandra?" she said simply.

"Yes, Mother," he replied, and it was done.

φ

"All right," said the Captain. "I have questions, difficult questions, about that first form of self-control: about not harming anyone."

"Roll ahead," I smiled.

"Is it only harming *others* that creates a bad seed? What if you harm *yourself?*" he began.

"Something like ... like trying to commit suicide?" I asked.

"Exactly," he said.

"The main point of not harming anyone is to avoid doing any damage to that incredibly rare and precious vehicle that we ride in: our body. In its current condition it is either a wreck already or a wreck waiting to happen, but—simply put—we really need it right now ... "

"So we can do what we need to, to plant the right seeds, to see it change into something that's *not* a wreck," he surmised.

"Exactly," I said. "And so knowingly doing harm to your own body—or to your mind, for that matter—plants very powerful negative seeds. We must be as kind to ourselves as we are to others."

Here the Captain paused, and then said, "It's not here on the list of questions," and I saw he had actually written himself out reminders of what to ask, "but it's something practical I need to know."

"Nothing's more practical than ideas," I said, "but go ahead."

"It's ... it's about the Sergeant," he went on. "I need to know ... are there any poses—any special ways of breathing or doing the silent sitting—that would be especially effective to help someone like him, help him stop hurting himself, with the alcohol?"

I nodded. "It's a common problem—not just with alcohol, but with any other kind of compulsive behavior, you see—people's lives taken over and controlled by just about anything: drinking, drugs, eating, smoking, sex, talking too much, doing too much. And the answer is that the best thing you can do is just take him through the very same thing we've been doing together: a short, but *very regular* daily practice of the poses; basic but *very regular* daily breathing exercises; and brief but *very regular* daily sitting, silently: taking away the same problem say from others, and sending them happiness, all upon the breath.

"You see, with yoga as we've talked about it, this regular modest daily practice causes very profound changes at the level of the channels and the inner winds. And that has a matching effect on the thoughts and attitudes themselves. Any person who just keeps this up steadily, a little each day, just naturally begins to avoid these bad habits—because these simply don't fit any more into who they are. And then one day they just naturally drop the habit completely: no big announcements or resolutions. They may not even notice."

The Captain nodded his thanks, and went on with his questions. "But . . . about this suicide thing . . . what if the person is in a lot of pain? What if life has become unbearable? And who cares about seeds, if you're about to die?"

I looked at him gravely, and felt Katrin's cold steel flowing into me. I searched desperately for a metaphor he could relate to.

"You have a house. It has only two rooms, and one door to the outside. You are in the room with the door to the outside. There is a friend with you. And in the room there are twenty small children running around, playing a game and screaming.

"Your friend has a very bad headache. He says he cannot bear it anymore. You say you will let him out the front door, but it happens to be locked. You ask him to hold on while you find the key.

"He says no, he truly can't bear it any longer, and he will go instead to the second room. But you know that inside that second room there is a dog, a savage dog, of immense size. And it is desperately hungry. And you know that it will rip your friend to pieces the moment he enters that room."

I stopped and fixed my eyes coldly on the Captain. He shifted uncomfortably on his seat, and finally looked up. "It's hardly a good example," he said then, a little defensively. "I mean, I suppose you're saying that . . . we must go on somewhere . . . after we die. But personally I cannot believe that, and—no matter what they say—I don't think many other people do either. We see people . . . we see them die. The body stops, and is still, and the life seeps out and they lie there—cold, dead. It's all over. We can see that it's all over."

A sort of anger came into me, hot now like Katrin too. "I will put it to you bluntly, Captain. The one and only reason that people think we don't go on after the body stops is—well—just that: they can see that the body has stopped. But if you are completely honest with yourself for even a single moment, you must say that you cannot be sure that the person's mind has stopped just because their body has stopped. Because when the body stops then the mind can no longer send any messages to the outside: no hands to wave, no tongue to speak with, no eyes even to blink. And so the whole world believes—really believes it, whether they admit it or not—that the person and the person's mind have stopped, with no better proof than a body that no longer moves. It's like saying a person riding in a coach must be dead, if the coach breaks a wheel and stops. It's exactly the same thing, let's be honest. At least admit that *you're not sure* if the mind goes on, to someplace else."

The Captain shook his head once, curtly, and looked down. I could feel he was starting to get a little upset. "But the wild dog thing; I mean, come on, fire and brimstone and all that."

Fire came into me then, but I struggled to hold it back, because I really didn't want him to be upset. I simply wanted him to be aware, aware of the dangerous power of seeds.

"Captain, please, look at your life—look even at just your life today. You got up, out of bed: you woke up. Thousands upon thousands of images flashed before you—*your world*—as you dressed, and ate breakfast, and walked to the station for just another normal day at work. And it was life as usual: nothing tremendously happy, nor tremendously painful either.

"But you see, just to maintain the flow of reasonably pleasant images—the toast at breakfast, the feel of the morning air, the touch of your own body, the song of your own thoughts—just to maintain what you take as normal life, it requires many thousands of seeds ripening instant after instant, presenting each detail of each object around you to your mind *instant by instant*. And these are all *good* seeds, you see, the very cream of all the countless seeds you've planted in your mind.

"And we use them up like that, you see—unknowingly, unaware, not even guessing at how many kind and wonderful actions we did towards others to create these seeds. And so the store of good seeds dwindles—which is WHY WE GROW OLD. And then when they are gone completely WE CALL IT DEATH, which we see as ourselves dying, when new seeds wake up. And these new seeds . . . " How to say it to him? How to say it so he would *see*? I couldn't think of anything but the blunt truth of it.

"Captain, we are awake for, say, 16 or 18 hours a day: for about a thousand minutes. Throughout the day, we purposely do or speak or think something kind to others—I mean *really* kind, and *purposely*—only, what? Five, ten, fifteen times, maybe half an hour, total? And then most of the rest, especially in our private thoughts, is spent viewing others in a critical way, in a judgmental way, in a competitive way—wrapped in a daze of selfishness.

"And so if we *do* go on, somewhere, after death—and you really cannot prove that we do not—then we go on with a storehouse of seeds which are almost all negative. I'm not saying that some big evil spirit has run around the world building invisible little rooms with big bad dogs in them. There is no such thing. I'm saying that—*if* the thing with the pen is right, and you know it is—then the seeds that every one of us carries to our death are certainly enough to *see*, to make us *be* in, places infinitely more painful than the most hopeless shred of life in this world. And so we must not kill—we must never even dream of killing—others or ourselves."

The Captain was silent for a long tense moment, and then sighed heavily. I felt tense myself. I am the teacher; I must say these things, even if he doesn't want to hear them, even if he thinks they're stupid, or wrong. A student is like a mother's child; the teacher is like a mother. Could a mother ever let her child open the door to that second room, without . . . without at least *trying* to give warning?

He glanced down at his list, tense.

"What about animals?" he said. "What about hurting, or killing, animals?"

"When the Master says not to harm *anyone*, he is referring to animals as well. You see, in the ancient languages, the words 'anyone' and 'person' refer to animals too: to anything that is conscious, anything with feelings."

"But animals don't have feelings," he replied curtly, something I guess he had heard an adult say when he was young.

"Then why . . . why did you scratch my dog's ears, that night . . . that night at your home?" I was beginning to feel strained myself.

"Oh, well . . . well, I mean, maybe . . . well obviously, *some* animals, like pets and so on—they obviously have feelings; that's what makes it so fun to take care of them: they respond with so much affection, you see. But I mean, you know—animals like, like fish say."

"And have you never stood at the banks of the river and seen a fisherman set that cruel steel hook in the mouth of a fish and struggle to bring him in, as the fish fights with his last strength to escape, even flying out of his own world to the air in which he cannot live, from the pain of it? How can you say he's not *feeling* anything?"

The Captain's face reddened. "Well, I mean that, yes, but—you know, all those smaller animals—so . . . so insignificant, in a way—and so obviously stupid."

The fire got hotter in me. "Babies . . . human babies . . . are small, and stupid too, you see. It makes them . . . defenseless, really. And it is the small ones, the defenseless ones, that *deserve* never to be the objects of our harm. Your own heart tells you that; I don't need to say it. It is humankind's one most glorious trait, that we feel the urge to protect those who are weak, and defenseless."

The Captain let out another, sharper sigh. I didn't know what to do. Perhaps I don't have enough experience to be teaching all these things to someone. Perhaps I should ask him to find a better teacher, an older one—someone who can explain all this without making him angry.

"And *plants?*" he asked tersely.

"The ancient books are clear in saying that plants are not *sentient* life—not like humans or animals. Plants respond to nutrients and grow, but the ancient books say more like the way that crystals do, and not with conscious life or feelings. And so we cannot harm them in that sense.

"These same books though are quite clear to say that we should *respect* plants, and do our best not to damage or destroy them without compelling need. This is because they provide homes for countless smaller creatures."

The Captain rolled his eyes. "Captain, sir, I am just trying . . . " but then I thought it better just to go on; perhaps we could reach a quiet point later where I could tell him I didn't mean to upset him.

He looked at his list again. "You mentioned babies," he said, sounding a little aggressive now. "What about . . . what about a baby in the womb—what about a fetus?"

This one was easy; so clear in all the ancient books. "Do you remember," I began, "when we spoke about how a baby forms, in the womb?"

He nodded stiffly. "I do: the flesh and bones form around the pattern of the subtle channels, like layers of ice around the contours of a twig. And so even the major joints that begin to pain us later in our lives have formed around knots in the channels that were there as early as the womb. But how early? "

I nodded, and took it straight from the ancient sources. "When the sperm of the father meets the egg of the mother— in that first instant—then something we call a *bindu* enters at that same moment: a spark of consciousness, a pin-point of awareness—one of those 'stars' that the Master spoke of. And then this pin-point of awareness begins to move, and the first channels begin to sprout, and as they do the first cell splits for the first time. And so there is consciousness, a very basic form of awareness, and life, even in the first moment. And it is, again, defenseless life, and it deserves our kindness and care all the more."

The Captain reached out and took his pen in his fingers and squeezed it tightly. His knuckles went white against the flesh. Not a good sign. My mind raced to think of ways to make him happy with me again. In that moment it felt more important than . . . than *teaching* him really.

He glanced one last time at his little list and then tossed it down on the table with something bordering on disgust. "War," he said. "The King starts a war, say.

"Now I understand the part about what I should do myself, already. I mean, if someone is hurting someone else, we must try to restrain them—without violence, and without hatred: without starting The Circle spinning back on us one more time. That much we've already talked about. But let's say that even if I don't go to fight the enemy myself, I support the war effort—let's say even just by paying my taxes.

"Now my question is this: if a soldier on the front line then kills someone, do *I* have any *part* of a seed planted by this in *my* mind—say, just because I helped pay for it?"

I nodded, eager to satisfy at least one of his questions easily. The ancient books were quite clear on this as well. "A lot of how seeds are planted depends on your motivation: your intention. If you really didn't *want* to support a war effort but you were compelled by law to pay taxes that ultimately *contributed* to that effort, then yes some small negative seeds would be planted, even in your own mind.

"If however you went further and made an effort to inform the authorities that you did *not* support your taxes being used to do violence towards others—if you worked earnestly, and honestly, and without violence to discourage that violence—then you would plant very *good* seeds in your mind.

"But if you in your mind—without thinking of the tremendous pain done to anyone on either side who lost a son or daughter, or even just a home or their crops—if you as you went through your daily life thought about the war sometimes vaguely and felt that it was all right; well then, the ancient books are very clear. If a single person dies, in a single remote battle, it is exactly as if you had stood before them with a knife and plunged it into their heart yourself. That kind of seed is planted in your own mind. And that kind of pain comes back to you, infinitely greater, when the evil tree has grown from that evil seed."

The Captain held the pen up, and then actually threw it across the room. My heart was pounding. I didn't know what to do. I began to wish that maybe we had just done some poses, and had a good sweat together. This wasn't the way I wanted it to be between us. I really felt very close to him.

"Too much!" he cried. "It's too much! I mean, these ideas of yours . . . "

"Not *mine*," I began to protest.

"No matter!" he cried. "These ideas—I can't accept them. I mean, they go against . . . they go against what, well, just what *everybody* knows; and what everybody says. And some of them, they are just, you know, *old-fashioned*, I mean. Modern thinking has gone way beyond them. They are quaint, in a way; they are, you can say, they are *good-hearted*, and *well-intended*. But they just aren't up to the level of thinking which is *current*; which is *sophisticated*; which is the result of the constant refinement and sensibilities of our whole society, here in the Realm, for the past *six hundred years!*" he proclaimed.

My head was starting to spin, but then a voice came to me, from inside: the voice of the Master. It calmed me and I repeated out loud what it told me. "On this, Captain, the Master says:

> *These various forms of self-control*
> *Are mighty codes of conduct*
> *Meant for people in every stage*

Of their personal development.
They go beyond
Differences in race or social status;
They go beyond
The borders between countries;
They go beyond
What is modern, or old;
They go beyond
The various creeds and convictions.

II.31

The Master is saying, you see, that what we do to help or to hurt others is at the bottom of everything: nothing works, not yoga or any other thing we ever do at all, unless we have been careful to plant the seeds in our mind to see it work. And he says, he says this one thing especially, with such passion—it is obviously the core of yoga, for the great father of all yoga; the core of all he ever says."

The Captain's face went tight; his mouth was a thin taut line of tension. And then he blurted out, "I don't know if I really *care* what the Master says."

My face snapped back as if he had slapped it. My mind went cold, and my heart hurt. But then the corporal came and saved us.

34

Worldview

Fourth Week of October

If we have been trying very hard to plant good seeds in our minds, slowly and steadily, for a while—then sometimes we get a glimpse of what life will be like in the end, and a little miracle comes to help us.

And so just at the one most difficult moment of my life in the jail, there was a little commotion outside the window; I felt the magic, and I clasped the Captain's hand in my own and pulled him up to see what it was, before he had a chance to think about it.

The corporal was there sitting in the dust like a little boy, the bottom of his white cotton pants getting all brown. Around him stood a little cluster of insistent sparrows, rushing in little groups to small pieces of his mother's flatbread as he tossed them around in a circle. His face was alive with a childlike joy at their happiness.

And we stood and watched, the Captain and I, at the window—our hands still touching, and the tension flowing away. The sunlight poured in happily and caught our faces, and I saw his handsome features relax at the corporal's lovely innocence. The little birds pulled at pieces of the bread, chirping furiously, as if they were playing tug-of-war. And then beautiful little red birds like finches landed and ended the little sparrow tussles, chasing away both sides and grabbing the pieces themselves. They were followed by larger squawking jays that did the same to the finches, and finally two huge black crows swooped down and sent everyone else on their way, devouring all the bread the corporal had. And he laughed and got up happily, and dusted off everything except a big round circle of brown centered over his backside, and walked slowly off out of sight, to the porch.

The Captain turned to me—the touch had healed us and gone—and said gently, "I'm sorry I got upset. You know I really do have a great respect for the Master, and for everything you have spoken of. It's just that . . . sometimes it's hard, when he says something that sort of goes against a lot of what you grew up with. It takes time . . . to think it over, to figure it out . . . "

I nodded. "It was the same for me, when my Teacher first introduced a lot of these ideas to me. I daresay I was much more stubborn than you are, much more set in my view of the world, even so young."

And then the crows took off into the air with their sharp loud caws, and I looked at the tiny crumbs of bread in the dirt; and the sparrows who had been there first began to hop back for whatever they could salvage.

"Sometimes I wonder," I said quietly, leaning my elbows on the window sill.

"Wonder what?" he said, leaning out next to me, and we drank the fresh air.

"I mean, look at life—look at just the way life works with the birds. Each one is absolutely intent on getting a piece of the bread for himself. And there is a natural order of things, you see: if you have the bread but if I show up and I'm bigger and stronger than you, then I simply take it away from you. And the same if someone bigger and stronger than me shows up—and that's just the way it goes.

"And that's how people have lived too; I mean most people, for as long as there have been people. But then you have to imagine that there was a day, long ago—somewhere, say maybe in a cave or something when humans first began. And one human comes in with maybe some berries or a little dead animal he has found, and he sits down to eat it.

"But then he sees that there's already another human there in the cave; and there's a tense moment while the two look each other over to see who's bigger and stronger: I mean, who will take the food from the other.

"And then something odd comes into the first one's mind, and he takes his berries or whatever and just hands some of them, or maybe all of them, over to the other person—without a struggle, without a fight; just because he *feels* how hungry the other one is.

"And then maybe the next day the first human goes out again looking for some food, and he is special, you see, and he notices that food *seems a lot easier to find* that day. And then some unspeakably holy, sacred string of thought passes through his mind and he says to himself, 'Maybe food is easier to find for me today because I shared my food yesterday.'"

I felt excited just thinking about that first glint of understanding, and I felt it begin too in the Captain at my side. "You see," I went on, looking into his face. "You see, he doesn't have any idea about seeds or pens or mental images forming because of a kindness he saw himself do before. He just has a flash of insight; he is framing in that moment the greatest invention that humankind has ever created: kindness.

"And you see, it's not just an instinct with him anymore at that moment. I mean he's not like an animal feeding its own young, or anything like that. He is moving up to a whole new level of humanity: a whole new evolution in the human spirit. Because he is beginning to undertake kindness *as a principle:* as part of the way he sees the world work. *He is showing kindness to another being because his very view of reality is changing:* he is developing this *new* worldview, where he grasps that the very *things and events around him* may be *created by the kindness he shows to others.*

"And at some point this worldview graduates to an even higher evolution: he sees not only that he can fulfill his own needs with this way of viewing his world; he sees that everyone else could fulfill *their* needs this way too, if he simply passes on to them what he has learned. Sharing his discovery of how kindness changes things, as he first shared his food.

"And so I guess you could call that moment the birth of yoga, or whatever name you may call this divine understanding of kindness and the sharing of kindness, in your own language and culture.

"And you see," I breathed to him, "This is all I meant to say today. This kind of thing—the human discovery of kindness—it goes beyond all differences in people or countries or times. And like all discoveries, like all great ideas, it can get lost for a while, in any one particular culture. Cultures—civilizations—they are just like individual people. They may be doing very well on the whole, good on a large scale, but then—just like any one of us—they might make a mistake, make a mistake as a whole people."

I sat him back down at the desk, but I took his hand again in my own, to make what I had to say easier. "I mean,

I will give you an example—it's just one example. And it may be hard for you, but I don't mean it to be—I just want it to be something you won't forget."

The Captain agreed with his eyes, warm and moist. It must be the same for anyone in the world who imagines the very discovery of kindness—especially kindness wrapped in real understanding.

"There is a young man, say," I began. "He grows up in the countryside and then comes to the city to find his career. And he manages to get a job in an office somewhere, and there are other young men working there—young men from the city itself.

"And then one evening they take him out to dinner, say, and they serve him some liquor. And he is watching all of them and there is this kind of ritual about the liquor: the waiter comes and flourishes it, the bottle is opened grandly, and immediately there is a kind of excitement and anticipation among his fellows.

"And rounds are poured for everyone, and downed, and he drinks his too—even though it just tastes to him like some terrible soup of rotten wheat or something. But it seems to be the thing to do, and he goes along with it, to fit in; and after some time he gets used to the taste.

"And he finds out at some point that it really is just the waste water from rotten grains or fruits, but that people in the city consider it quite important and sophisticated, even arguing between them whether the waste water from one rotten grain is more 'smooth' or more 'mellow'; or whether barley rotted for a few months in copper kettles tastes better than grapes rotted for a few years in wooden barrels; things like that.

"And to him they all taste pretty much the same—just the taste of something that has spoiled—but he doesn't let on, because you see this liquor thing seems like something that people who live in the city should know about and use constantly: it has an aura of romance, or adventure, or kinship; something. And so he learns to drink, and the people around him teach him to drink, simply by their example.

"And then one day someone close to the young man dies, you see, and he has this tremendous pain that never lets up, even for a moment, even at night for sleep. And he finds out that if he drinks a lot of the rotten water then the pain is numbed for a few hours. And then the drinking grows and grows, and it gradually takes over his life, and then it gets ugly, and the very people who taught him to drink don't want anything to do with him.

"And then gradually you see his own life is ruined, and for the sake of any companionship at all he draws others into his drinking, and then . . . perhaps . . . even one day . . . he drinks too much and then causes an accident, and someone—someone very innocent—is hurt, hurt seriously. And then on that day he wakes up, and he realizes something: that this liquor thing, this adventure and ritual of the fine drink, it was all . . . simply . . . one horrible, useless tragedy; a simple and terrible mistake in the path his life has taken."

The Captain's head was bowed with the pain of remembering it all. I squeezed his hand tight and brought his eyes back up to mine.

"And so you see, there are things—there are ways of behaving, there are ways of viewing the things around us—that a person as he or she goes through their life simply discovers are a mistake. And they discover it the hard way. And people—real people, good honest people—they get hurt, they get hurt sometimes in a way that can't be fixed.

"And on a larger scale, whole countries—whole cultures, whole civilizations even—they can make mistakes the very same way as an individual person can. I mean, the liquor is a good example. What is it really? Just an accident: good honest food like barley or wheat that could have been made into bread to fill the bellies of the poor, and the children of the poor, who are always with us—and this food is left somewhere to rot, to spoil. And then a whole network of mystique takes it over and packages it and sells it and serves it and makes it seem exciting and sophisticated. And then it goes into people's bodies and a great many of them can't control themselves and gradually it causes them great illness and sadness, a sadness that spreads and poisons the lives of their wives and husbands and children.

"And the culture, you see—the viewpoint they grew up with, about liquor: that it's something exciting, something that will bring companionship or romance into their lives— this viewpoint will survive the ones who are destroyed by it. And so the culture—which is really just a big group of people over lots of generations—has been infected by a *viewpoint*, by a *way of viewing the world*, which not only doesn't help the people who *are* the culture, but actually does them great harm. These same viewpoints though, you see, can be strong once they get started.

"And that's because of the way they are passed down from one generation to the other. I mean, most of our viewpoints about say harming other beings are not something that we in any way came up with on our own. Almost everything we *do*, and almost everything we *believe* in, we do or believe in for one reason, and for one reason only: it is what our parents taught us; it is what we learned from an older brother or sister; it is what the teachers in the school said when we were very small; it is—*it is what everyone else does*. It is what everyone *else* believes. AND THEY ARE ONLY DOING OR BELIEVING IN IT BECAUSE SOMEONE ELSE DID BEFORE THEM, and for no better reason.

"And so you see, a very bad way of acting—a very bad way of *thinking* about things—it can just keep itself going, blindly, madly, from generation to generation, like the myth of 'fine liquor.' The Master is talking about this when he says,

> *The sixth obstacle*
> *Is a mistaken view of the world*
> *Left uncorrected.*
>
> I.30F

I mean, liquor is just a small example. There are other worldviews which can simply destroy an entire civilization, unnoticed. The idea that war could end violence. The idea that the number of things you have in your house, or the *size* of your house, could even remotely make you happier. The idea that you *obtain* things by competing aggressively with *others* who want those same things, and not by doing *the exact opposite*.

"The idea that you must die. The idea that you must grow older. The idea that a body made of pure light in a perfect world of light is only a fairy tale, only some old myth, and not something real that you can reach simply by undertaking a very simple and sincere series of very practical steps, as we are doing now.

"And so the great Masters of old, you see, wherever they have lived around the world, they have taught their people to follow the code of self-control. And before it was a rule it was a *code*, a *personal* code: a way of life that you kept from the inside, and not because someone outside told you you had to. You followed it because you knew it would put seeds in you that would create a perfect body and mind to carry into a perfect world. And you knew that if you could do it yourself, then you could really help others do it.

"And so here is where the Master grants us the great gift of the highest form of self-control of all. It is not the act of avoiding harm to our body or the bodies of others. It is not anything that we say, kind or cruel. It is *how we see things*, for this view of the world—this *worldview*—is what will determine what all of us do in our words and actions, and what we pass on to our children for *them* to follow.

"And he says finally that we must be willing, for the sake of others and the children who come after us, to *examine* how we view the world. To *think about* what we have learned from all those around us and all who came before us, and see if it is really *helpful*. See if it *really works the way everyone said it did*. Or perhaps see that it *does not work at all*, and *never did*: like the lie of liquor. And if we discover that a worldview does not work—if it does not help people, if it does not really bring real happiness to people—then we must have the courage to *stop* following it, and *correct* it, and not blindly pass on to our children something which *will not work for them either*, something which may even *hurt* them.

"And so what I mean, Captain, is that I am offering you new ideas. A new way of viewing the world: a new way of understanding *how things really work*, and how we can stop even the grand mistakes of unhappiness, the aging of the body, and death itself. But you must listen with an open mind; a mind opened by the realization that the way we were taught to view the world *simply doesn't work* on these most important points of our life.

"And if the new viewpoint doesn't seem to make sense, then you must ask questions about it until you are satisfied, or else you should wait on it, or even reject it too, and continue with your search elsewhere. But if you examine these ideas, this new most ancient worldview, and you find that they *do* make sense, then you must have the courage to give them a good try, for your own sake and for the sake of others. And that is something," I drew myself up tall as Katrin would have, "*much different* from throwing your pen across the room every time you are presented with an idea that is new to you, but which may very well actually save your life, and the lives of all you care for."

I stopped finally but kept hold of his hand. He was just staring into my face, mesmerized again by the real possibilities that were opened up. The dream of a perfect world is too strong to die in our minds, even after we cross the border into adulthood. It just needs waking up sometimes.

He nodded silently, solemnly, and we went and did our giving and taking, and our breathing, and knocking on the pipes with our good old sweaty poses.

φ

"We've got to get all this organized before it gets completely out of control," announced the Sergeant. He was talking to Busuku and me face-to-face, huddled in a little trio on the floor of my cell. Busuku and I were too surprised to do anything more than just listen to him as he went on intensely.

"I mean, there's just too many people involved now to let it go on haphazardly," he continued, oblivious to our uncomprehending stares. "Now as I see it, first priority is Miss Friday's weekly class with the Captain, since the Captain has to turn around and pass those onto the corporal and myself right afterwards. So that should take place, say, on Monday mornings, as early as possible." He looked up at the window. "I'll inform the Captain," he said, and made a note on a little piece of paper before him.

"Now my boy Ajit should be coming in say right after that, since children are so much more fresh before noon. That means you'll have to get your boys in by mid-morning too, Busuku . . . " Busuku's incomprehension deepened noticeably. "That is, if this fits in with Miss Friday's weaving schedule," and the Sergeant looked at me, but I was catching as little of this as Busuku—who finally stirred himself.

"Ravi, what on earth do you mean about my boys? What do they have to do with all this?" he demanded.

"Ah, that," rushed on the Sergeant, hardly even pausing. "I was home last night thinking about the Captain's last class with Miss Friday . . . " Here he reddened a bit, but Busuku saved him.

"Oh, I get it!" exclaimed Busuku, his face alive with his thoughts. "Oh, brilliant, Ravi. You're going to put that worldview thing into practice right away. Break out of that idiot worldview of taking care of just ourselves: the worldview that everyone drilled into us growing up. Taking care of the other boys too, so you can see the yoga work on them *and* your boy. The key to how yoga really works: the ultimate worldview, taking care of others. Atta boy, Ravi!" and he gave the Sergeant a hearty slap on the back that set him to choking.

Then to me Busuku winked and said, "Oh, that was a great last class with the Captain, Miss Friday. We were all eavesdropping and cheering you on. Ravi said he was going to go in and plow those new worldview seeds into the Captain's head with his stick, if he ever threw his pen across the room again—didn't you Ravi?"

And Busuku slapped the Sergeant again on the back, which set him to choking again, and whispered to me: "Seeds! Ripening! From smacking you and me before, you see! And I'm just *helping them ripen!*" And he slammed the Sergeant's back one last time, for good measure.

When he had mostly recovered, the Sergeant went on, shifting a bit out of Busuku's range without even thinking. "And then Miss Friday, what I see is a quick lunch for you—we'll see that you get a nice proper dinner later in the evening—and then the class with the corporal's mother; I guess three days a week would be enough to start?" I nodded dumbly, overwhelmed by it all.

"Good! Then it's all decided!" He stood quickly and tapped Busuku lightly on the head with the end of his stick. "Now back to your cell, Rotund One! I need a few words with Miss Friday privately."

Busuku worked himself up with a groan—"I can't believe you made me do the Longbow Pose *three* times last night," he moaned at me—and shuffled off to his cell. "And don't forget again to come and bar my door," he yelled back at the Sergeant. "People walk in and look at me funny, like I'm too dumb to escape, you know," he whined.

The Sergeant squatted down next to me again. "I really want to thank you for Ajit," he began, and he almost started to cry, which did start me crying. "He is so much happier, and he hasn't been able to walk this well in years, not since . . . " I nodded quickly; it needn't be said.

"And he asks . . . he asks me to ask you . . . if you would let him take Long-Life out for walks, you see. Say once in the morning, and once in the evening. He says . . . he says he thinks he has figured out . . . a way . . . " and the Sergeant stopped again, laughing almost crying, " . . . a way to make Long-Life's legs all better—some kind of yoga poses for puppies that Ajit says he's worked out during his silent sitting at home."

I nodded. "That would be wonderful; wonderful for Long-Life, wonderful seeds for Ajit," I said.

"Then that's decided too," said the Sergeant, checking his paper once more and then folding and slipping it into his shirt pocket. On the way out the door he turned and said, "Ajit has also offered to give Long-Life a bath—say, once a week. That way he won't be bringing in any fleas."

"Fleas?" I said.

"I mean, yes . . . fleas. I don't want a dog staying in one of our cells and bringing fleas . . . " My mouth dropped open.

"In, or out!" smiled the Sergeant, and he strolled out to the front porch, into the sunlight.

35

Matching Pictures

First Week of November

"On to the second form of self-control!" I announced—to the Captain, and to the back of the door, and to the mud wall on the other side. Actually, I thought, it was a pretty efficient way of teaching three classes at once. The Captain looked at me eagerly. I could tell he'd been thinking things over hard; the rightness of it all had touched him in deep places, and given him hope to replace the doubt. Then suddenly his forehead wrinkled a bit, and I knew there was a question, and I nodded for it to come.

"It's about the caveman," he began slowly.

I nodded again.

"I mean," he went on, "you talk about him discovering kindness, and I understand that, and it's truly an inspiration.

"But then I was thinking about it, and it began to seem to me that he was being kind to others not because it would help *them*, but because it would help *himself*. And to tell you the truth, that doesn't set right in my heart."

I nodded a third time. It was a common concern, and a very valid one.

"There's something here you have to realize," I began, "and then it will come clear. You see, it's not a question of my happiness *or* others' happiness, although our minds are often setting it up that way. If you are really committed to helping others reach some kind of ultimate happiness—if that is what you live for—then in the end of all ends you will come to realize that you can only do so by reaching this happiness yourself, so that then you can come back and show them how to do it.

"And — here is where the seeming paradox comes in— you can only reach your own happiness if you are already doing it for others. So this is how it works: you want to help others to be happy; so you work towards that happiness yourself; wanting to help others lets you reach it; and then you are in a position to carry out what you wanted in the first place: to bring others there."

He gazed up and thought for a while, and then looked back down at me with a smile. "What you're saying," he concluded, "is that no one can be happy unless everyone is, and that everyone won't be happy until one is." He paused then and added, "Or, you can say, that we can't leave ourselves out when we undertake to make the whole world happy." Another pause. "Because *we* are part of the whole world too!" And he grinned brightly.

"You've got it," I smiled back, and we started on again. "Now the Master says that

> *The second form of self-control*
> *Is always telling the truth.*
>
> II.30B"

"That's pretty clear," said the Captain, in that voice that said, "Well actually, you know, I almost never lie."

I gazed at him thoughtfully. "You know, most of us," I said slowly, "we sort of think we already don't do so badly with all these different kinds of self-control.

"But there's a difference between, you see, sort of a socially acceptable level of self-control—the amount of self-control we all show to each other anyway, in an amount that prevents the world from being a total madhouse all the time—and the degree of self-control we have to cultivate in ourselves if we ever hope to see a major change in the seeds we are creating.

"I mean, think of a cow setting out on the task of turning a stick which is something to eat into a pen whose existence and function is almost totally beyond her comprehension, and then you get a very good feeling for our own efforts to plant seeds in our minds so powerful that they change our entire physical and mental being to the level of pure and angelic creatures. Possible, but difficult. Our efforts at self-control have to become a constant song within us, that we sing as we pass through every moment of the day.

"And with telling the truth, this means that it's not enough simply not to tell frequent, blatant lies. I mean, that much we avoid already and—and it has *not* been enough to alter our very reality. Truth for us now has to reach a deeper level; and the ancient books say that this means *striving, as we speak*, never to create even the smallest misimpression in the mind of the person listening to us.

"The picture *they* get in their mind after we say what we have to say must *match*, as closely as we can get it to match, the picture we ourselves have in our mind already about the thing we are speaking of. The closer these two pictures match is *truth*. Any difference created on purpose between the two pictures is *lying:* enough of a lie so that we would never, say, see a person come into our lives and explain to us how yoga really works."

The Captain frowned ever so slightly, and stared at his desk, and then at the piles of reports stacked—more neatly now—around his seat. "Now that's a lot more difficult than simply not lying . . . " he began.

"No, it's what it *really* means not to lie," I contended.

"Ah yes," he said, slowly. "I suppose . . . I suppose that's right; it doesn't take a lot of thought to see that." And then he considered a moment longer. "But it seems like it would be extremely difficult to reach and maintain that level of honesty," he said frankly.

"At first," I admitted. "But people are funny that way, you see. We can get used to anything, if we really try. You just start small and steady, and then you build up. I mean, you and I can both imagine a society where this level of truthfulness is simply the norm that everyone lives by, because they have been trained that way from childhood, and the whole culture supports and expects and rewards total honesty. In the end it's just a habit, like anything else. And if we truly consider the rewards—say, escape from the effects of old age, and even death—then there is certainly enough incentive that we could do it if we really tried."

I felt then the Captain feeling the immensity of the effort though, especially since we were both already in a culture that would *not* support us much if we really tried this new level of honesty. And so I decided to tell him about the book, then and there.

"There's a way you can do it," I said. "It's a way that has been taught for thousands of years. You see, in the old days—even before paper—people who wanted to learn to keep these different forms of self-control on a very fine level would go out say to the bank of a river and collect a good-sized handful of smooth pebbles. Half the pebbles would be white, and half would be black. Just *little* pebbles, you see—about the size of a pea.

"They'd keep these pebbles say in a little bag, and they'd keep that and another, smaller pouch with them all day. And then if they caught themselves telling even a small lie or something like that they'd right away reach in and take a black pebble out of the bigger bag and put it in the little pouch.

"If on the other hand they did something to protect life, say—maybe showed someone how to do a yoga pose—or anything else that was good, well then they'd stop and put a white pebble in with the black one. And then at the end of the day they'd empty out the little pouch, count the white and black pebbles, and see if they'd taken a step ahead or a step back in trying to fill their mind with good seeds.

"And nowadays the way we do it is say just carry a little notebook around with us in a pocket, and three times a day—say before we eat—we pull it out and jot down the one best white seed we've planted in the last few hours, and the one worst black one. The ancient masters of yoga did this six times a day, and then at night before they went to sleep they looked over the list to see how they had done: take joy in the white seeds; and think about the black ones. And as they actually fell off to sleep they'd make plans for doing better on each when they got up the following morning.

"Because, you see, it's not enough say just to read a book that tells you how the yoga poses will never work for you if you're in the habit of hurting others or telling lies—even something like little white lies to your boss at work. You need a system that you can follow, every day all day, to actually get results.

"And that's what we call 'the book'; start today if you like, and review your day—pluses and minuses—at the very least do it once, before you sleep. Go through each of the five forms of self-control you will learn and make yourself a note about the best and the worst you did with each one. Stick to small, real and specific things that happened that day. And as you fall off to sleep plan your attack for the next day."

The Captain nodded once, with that military nod of his, and I knew he had caught it and would try it. But he also seemed distracted by something else, and his eyes kept wandering back to the stacks of reports.

Finally he said, "Now there's something that you said just now—you mentioned 'white lies to the boss at work.' But I have a problem with that, you see. Because, well, suppose you've made a mistake on a small project your boss has given you. And you know that in a day or two you could probably fix it, and no one would ever be the wiser. But then the boss comes and asks you whether there are any problems with the project he's given you. In a case like that—knowing he'd be angry with you if you said anything—wouldn't it be . . . wouldn't it be better . . . if you just told a little white lie?"

He looked up at me sheepishly, and I gave him that little pout of disappointment that I used to get from Katrin.

"Now Captain, I'm surprised at you. Of course you wouldn't want to tell a lie, even a 'little white lie.' And you tell me why."

The Captain fidgeted for a moment with his pen, trying to think how to avoid the obvious. And then a muffled cry came through the wall, from the back of the jail.

"*Doesn't work!*" it said.

"Shut up, Busuku!" burst out the Sergeant, sounding as if his ear were still glued to the door.

"*Culture mistake!*" yelled Busuku again.

"*Busuku!*" screamed the Sergeant.

"Civilization mistake!" roared Busuku, and then the Sergeant struck his stick hard on the floor three times, and complete silence ensued.

The Captain got red and then smiled. "But he's right, you know," he said quietly. "Busuku's right. If everything we're saying is true, it can't be that telling the truth to my boss would make him get angry at me. I mean, it's like the lie and the extra money: they may come one right after the other, and so the lie may *seem* to cause the extra money, but really a bad seed can't create a good result any more than the seeds from a thorn bush could grow into grape vines.

"And so here too a good seed—telling the truth—could never create a bad result: the boss getting angry at you. What Busuku is saying," continued the Captain, "is that lies—even little white lies—don't work. That is, they don't work *all the time*, which proves that if the boss *doesn't* get angry at me it's *not* because I fed him a white lie.

"And even the idea of a white lie—even the words *white lie*—they are just another mistake our whole culture has made, and made together. It is, as Busuku said so rightly, even a mistake that our entire civilization has made, century after century. And if I guess right, it is the seeds of mistaken ideas like this that throttle even a civilization's life in the end, in the same way that harmful actions we do towards others create the knots in our channels that make us as individuals get old and die."

I looked at my pupil with pride; now *he* was beginning to sound like Katrin. "And you *will* find," I said then, "that consistently being completely honest over an extended period of time *does* work; and *works all the time*. You will find that it creates an ever-higher upward spiral, where boss and fellow worker and family begin to honor and respect you for all that you say. And whatever old seeds you had to see people upset with you when you told the truth are eventually choked off themselves."

"There's a point there," interjected the Captain. "Is there any way to just *go after* old bad seeds like that, and get rid of them *before* they ripen into something unpleasant?"

"Later!" I smiled, but it was the most wonderful of questions. "Now a final point about honesty, before we get down to your poses." The Captain grimaced a bit, as does every student whose hopes of getting out of their daily work have been smashed.

"Since you are already teaching others, it's important that you know the most powerful kind of honesty there is. And that is always being careful to teach this knowledge of yoga—this oh so powerful worldview—exactly as you have learned it, never throwing in some idea that's occurred to you that you *think* might be right; never leaving out any of the important ideas that are *already* part of the tradition.

"Because, you see, the teachings on this way—the information in the Master's *Short Book*—they are like a list of instructions drawn up by a master physician to treat a person who has just been bitten by a deadly snake. The instructions have been written down by the best there is— *and they work.*

"Now suppose someone like you or me—someone even with a fair amount of training, and certainly with the best of intentions—comes along and begins throwing in unnecessary instructions, or even taking out necessary ones. Then what happens is . . . well, you know that party game for children where ten kids sit down in a row, and the first one whispers something to the second, and so on to the tenth, and then this last child says what he thinks he heard out loud, and it's always very funny because it's not at all what the first child whispered first.

"But here, with these instructions, it is no joke at all. They work, *as they were intended*; and *as they were written down*. And if we do not maintain a high level of honesty around them—that is, if we change them, or especially make claims about our own experiences with them that are not completely true—then we are already whispering *something different* into the next child's ear. And if the person we have whispered to is foolish enough to do the same, and so on down the line—then *at some point the instructions are changed so much that they no longer work*.

"And then someone who's been bitten by a snake—any one of the countless people alive now, or in the future, who are struggling to beat off the Lord of Death—they will *try* to practice the instructions as they have received them; and these instructions *will no longer work*. And so this seed, perhaps the most terrible seed of all, we must at all costs avoid."

36

Planting
Higher Seeds

Second Week of November

Teaching Mata Ji, the corporal's mother, was a real pleasure. She had it seems done some yoga in her early years, obviously with a person who really understood how yoga works. And so she came to her classes warm and open and ready to be taught.

Katrin had shown me a whole series of yoga poses that were especially good for older people; especially effective at loosening up bent and frozen joints in a way which was gentle, but which also quickly produced noticeable results for anyone as quietly dedicated as Mata Ji.

She also took to giving and taking in the silent sitting, like a fish to water; she took an obvious joy in rescuing people from their problems, and sending them their fondest hopes, all on her breath. It was this inner work on the channels I think that changed her hands so quickly.

When the Sergeant led Mata Ji into my cell for classes, he seemed increasingly embarrassed by the crossbar on the door. And then finally he just took the bar home one night and came back with it the next day, set it in its place, and called for me to have a look. Mata Ji and I had just finished a class.

"See how it works," he smiled. "Push on your door."

I did; the crossbar suddenly separated in two, and the door swung free.

"Took me a while to get it right, you see," he said proudly. "I sawed it here," he pointed to the edge of the door, "and then sanded it down, and then painted it all this matching color, you see.

"So if anyone comes and visits the jail unexpectedly— say, the *Superintendent*," and he raised his eyebrows, "then it will just look like a regular crossbar, you see. But for most days, well then you can just escort Mata Ji out to the front porch in a civilized manner, and no one has to feel . . . you know, like *locked in*."

I smiled at how little like a jail the jail was becoming, and the Sergeant and I tried out the door, to walk Mata Ji to the porch. She stepped out to the road and turned around and gave us a big wave, and we waved back with sunny smiles. Then the two of us stood at the rail enjoying the day, and something suddenly occurred to me.

"Sergeant, sir," I began, and he turned to face me, the sun still there in his smile.

"Yes, Miss Friday?"

"Sergeant, there is . . . there is something I've always wanted to ask you. I hope you won't find me . . . too forward . . . for asking."

"Why, go right ahead," he smiled on. "Anything at all, Miss Friday."

"Well you see, the Captain and I were talking once, a while back, and he . . . he mentioned something, just offhand."

"What's that?" said the Sergeant, gazing up at the sky with a look of contentment.

"Well, he said . . . I mean, do you remember the very first day, at the little guardhouse on the road?"

"Of course I do," he smiled. "It changed my life—changed all our lives."

"Yes, but, well—you see—the *Captain* said, and I don't know if that's exactly what he meant, you see, but he said that . . . that, well, you were actually *looking out for me* in the first place; that someone had actually *warned* you to look out for me."

The Sergeant turned back to me with a little look of surprise. "Well now that you mention it, yes—yes, we were told to keep an eye out for someone matching your description. Why, I'd forgotten about that altogether!"

"Well, yes, but . . . may I, Sergeant, may I ask . . . *who it was* that told you this?"

He gazed at me innocently and said, "Well of course, Miss Friday. It was . . . it was just Busuku, you see."

φ

"Third form of self-control!" I announced, and the Captain hunkered down with a serious look. I'd been worried about that.

"Captain, sir, don't look so serious!" And then I paused and added, "I hope you don't think I'm getting preachy or anything; I really don't mean to."

"Well," he admitted, "there are times when it reminds me of lectures on proper behavior that I used to get from my grandmother."

My face got red, and I felt flustered for a minute. "I guess it might sound like that sometimes," I said finally. "But it's . . . it's different, you see. I don't mean to sound like I'm telling you that you're a bad boy—like I'm telling you what you can and cannot do.

"I mean—I just want you to know, to know what the Master says are the few most powerful ways to plant good seeds. And the good seeds, you see, they're not like some kind of rules or obligations. It's not something you have to do, or something you're supposed to do. Good seeds are just, well, like regular seeds, that you plant in a garden. I'm just going over for you what the Master says are the easiest and strongest seeds you can plant to get the most wonderful lovely juicy watermelons you can imagine. Now once you've heard about them, it's really all up to you what you *do* about it."

The Captain nodded knowingly. "You are basically offering me a free ticket to create whatever beautiful thing I desire. I get that. I can put up with the occasional preachiness; I know where it's all going." Then he paused for a moment and added, "But the prospect of being able to bring about anything I wish for brings up an old question again."

"How's that?" I asked.

"I mean, a long time ago, you told me I should learn to overcome preferences. I believe we were . . . ah . . . referring to the Boat Pose, where you bust your guts, as opposed to the Dead Man's Pose, where you basically lie down and enjoy a nice, hard-earned rest."

"Yes," I said.

"And then later you said that liking some things and disliking other things was a big part in the chain of events that causes pain to come back to us again and again in a big, self-perpetuating Circle."

"Yes," I said calmly, as Katrin would have.

"And then somewhere in there you said it was *fine* to like some things and dislike other things."

"Yes," I said, still smiling.

"And now you've just reminded me that all this self-control stuff is really just part of a master plan to get me *whatever I want*."

I nodded yet again.

"Well, I even have a problem with *that*," he declared, and clacked his pen down firmly on the desk.

"How's that?" I said.

"What's the use of having things go your way for a while?" he said. "Everybody knows it's going to change again anyway. What's the use of even trying?"

"Ah, that," I said, and as usual it was a very fine question. But "First things first," I said.

"When I said not to get wrapped up with preferences," I said, "I was talking about *things that had already happened:* seeds that had already gone off in your mind. I mean, if someone serves you a meal and there are some things on the plate that you really enjoy and some that you don't care much for, but they are all types of food that are perfectly fine and healthy for you, well then you should go ahead and eat, ignoring your preferences; because this is what your seeds have brought to you at the moment, and it's too late to change them once they have ripened right *now*.

"And getting upset, you see—*that* would be falling into the kind of liking and disliking that causes all our pain, and keeps it going. Sometimes I like to call it *stupid* liking and *stupid* disliking. *Stupid* liking is looking at something you want and trying to struggle against others to get it. *Stupid* disliking is trying to get away from something you don't want even if you have to hurt someone to do so. Because neither one of these *works*, you see.

"If it *worked* to get you what you want, then maybe— just *maybe*—it would make sense to hurt someone else, or to tell a lie. But they *don't* get you what you want, because they don't *always* get you what you want, and so they *can't be* what really gets you what you want.

"And what *really* gets you what you want—WHAT ALWAYS WORKS TO GET YOU WHAT YOU WANT—is choosing what you want to happen and then very purposely planting the seeds that will *make* it happen later on. And these seeds always involve taking care of *others*. Which is why we're covering the ways we can slip up and *not* do things that are nice: because if we can do the *opposite* of these then we plant the best seed of all.

"And that brings us to *intelligent* liking, and *intelligent* disliking. Wish for anything you want—you *should* wish for anything you want—we *live* to fulfill all our wishes, great and small. But then go about *getting* it in the right way; which is to say, in the way that really *works:* in the *only* way that works. Plant the seeds—plant the right seeds; be a gardener—and then sit back and watch the fireworks."

"But what we *wish* for," urged the Captain. "*That's* the question. What's the use of planting seeds for *things that won't last?*"

"Oh yes," I said. "It's the same thing we spoke about that night at your home." He nodded gracefully; it was a pleasant memory for us both.

"The problem you're raising is covered first by the Master when he says,

> *The torment of change*
> *Is caused by these same*
> *Seeds of suffering.*
>
> II.15A

You see, on a deeper level, you're right; as you were that night at your house. Suppose someone has gotten too heavy and is hoping that doing yoga might be able to help them. And suppose that they meet up with a good teacher who not only knows all the best yoga poses for them, but also understands how yoga really works: they know that the poses will have to be targeted at the root of the problem—at blockages in the subtle channels; and they also know that this will only work if the person has collected the right seeds, by working very hard at being kind to others.

"And then say the whole process is successful, and the right seeds get planted—or woken up, if they are already there. And because of this the yoga poses themselves have the hoped-for effect on the inner channels, and the person through regular and continued practice is able to become slender, strong, and healthy again.

"And your question is—such a good question it is—why should we even *try* to become slender and strong? Because we all know that, sooner or later, it will change again—if nothing else, we will lose the slender, strong body itself as we grow older and older, and finally die.

"And what the Master is saying here is—yes, this is a problem. This is what we call the 'torment of change.' Bad seeds, well—no one needs to say—they are bad because they bring us obvious pain; they make us see obvious pain. But even good seeds too bring us their own pain: the pain of change, because whatever seeds we have planted by past goodness to others, and which now ripen and make us see ourselves slender and strong again, *wear out* simply *by* making us be slender and strong, for so many weeks or months.

"And then it's like we're thrown back to zero, which usually feels worse if we arrive at it fresh than if we'd simply always been there from before: say, if the weight problem had just stayed with us the way it was. It's the *change* that hurts the most.

"And so what the Master is saying, you see, is that *all* of the seeds really—good *or* bad—are 'seeds for suffering.' And I guess it's actually a good place — here in the middle of explaining self-control, the art of planting good seeds and avoiding bad seeds—that we explain how to plant *higher* kinds of good seeds: good seeds that *never wear out*."

The Captain nodded excitedly. "That's exactly what I was wondering about. I was hoping that there might be a kind of 'higher' good seed. Because in my heart—and I guess everyone else is the same really—I don't want to learn some way of making good things happen and then later on just have to face the same old disappointment as they begin to change, and fade away."

"Exactly," I said happily. He was so *good* at getting down into the middle of his own feelings and expressing his real thoughts about things.

"To put it simply, there *is* a way to plant *higher* good seeds, and I think we should go over it now that we're focused on it. And then we'll go on with the other forms of self-control at our next class—agreed?" The Captain smiled gratefully.

"Now the great books throughout time have said that you need two things to turn a regular good seed—one that will bring you something you hope for and then just wear out— into a *higher* good seed: one that will *never* wear out. The first thing you need, the first step you need to take, is described by the Master like this:

> *Use the eye of wisdom,*
> *Which comes from*
> *Mastering those three.*
>
> III.5"

"*What* eye of wisdom?" asked the Captain. "And *which* three?" he said with exasperation. "Why does the Master always sound like he's talking in code?"

I grinned with understanding. "I always wondered the same thing. And my Teacher used to say that, in the old days, everyone knew all these things already, and the book was just sort of a shorthand for remembering.

"The first step to planting a higher type of good seed in your mind is to look upon the good things you're doing with the 'eye of wisdom,' even as you do it. Let's say you've been working really hard on that form of self-control where you never harm anyone. And you're getting so *good* at it that now it's graduated into doing all sorts of great things on a daily level to *promote* other people's physical health and well-being. It's actually what you are doing already, say by teaching the yoga poses and ideas to the Sergeant and the corporal."

The Captain looked excited just remembering his students. There's nothing that feels more rewarding than passing all these things on to others once you've learned them yourself. And that's because of the tremendous seeds you plant as you pass them on, accurately.

"So let's say you've got the corporal sitting down on the floor in that Lord of the Fish pose, turned around to the back so he can work off that little belly from his mom's wonderful flatbread. The first thing you do is just *decide* you want this good seed planted as a higher good seed: you *focus* on this idea. This is the same practice of focus that we were talking about before, and it's the first of the 'three' that the Master just mentioned.

"Then you *concentrate* on what's going on. You *fix* your mind there; and this is the same 'fixation' we talked about before too. You *hold* your mind on the idea of making this good deed plant a *higher* seed. This is essential during the actual moments that the seed is being planted—while you're actually physically reaching out and helping the corporal with his pose—and also when you reflect back on it later and enjoy the good thing you did; which incidentally goes a long way in making the new seed *firm and strong*. This concentration or fixation is the second of the Master's 'three' here.

"And then lastly there is what the Master elsewhere calls 'perfect meditation,' which in this case is actually just thinking very hard, as you help the corporal, about what's really happening. I mean, Captain, you tell me . . . what would happen if, as you were sitting here helping the corporal with a pose, you suddenly began to remember very strongly that thing about the pen and the cow?"

The Captain turned his head and gazed out the window to collect his thoughts.

"Well, I suppose first of all that I'd think about how the yoga poses that the corporal was doing are really only sort of—neutral, I guess you could say. I mean, I guess I'd think about how *whether they worked for him* really depended on whether he had good seeds in his mind, that would ripen and change him, deep down at the level of his channels.

"And then I suppose that I'd think about the seeds *in my own mind* going off even as I watched the corporal. I mean, I'd know that really the whole *class* was sort of neutral or blank or what we called empty, in a way; but only in the sense that—if I happened to see the class work out successfully for the corporal—it would really only be because I had good seeds going off in my own mind, making me see something very good happening—something I had really *hoped* would happen."

"And so really," I said, "the *whole scene* would be imbued with an awareness of how things are not themselves until your own seeds make you see them that way. And focusing and fixing your mind on this meditation or line of thinking as the class goes on is an art in itself: if you get *good* at it—if you *master* it—then you have what we call the 'eye of wisdom.' You are looking at the class with the three parts of the eye of wisdom: focusing your thoughts; fixing them there; and then running through the idea of the pen and the cow, really.

"And the Master feels so strongly about these three that he devotes a great deal of his book to describing the powerful things you can do if you use them all together, frequently.

"He also gives them their own name, which we heard him mention way back in his description of the sun channel: he calls them the 'combined effort.' And over and over again he tells us how this 'combined effort' can plant higher good seeds: seeds so powerful that they cause a complete transformation in our own body, and our mind, and our entire world.

"And so there it is, the first step to planting a good seed that *won't* wear out. As you do good for others—as you do your gardening with the seeds in your own mind using kindness itself—then simply *think* about it, deeply: 'Everything I am seeing here is coming from seeds. And now by doing good, I consciously and purposely plant good seeds for a perfect future.' And simply the *understanding* of what you are doing *as you do it* transforms the very way it is planted.

"In terms of those subtle channels deep within us, you are planting seeds from the *middle* channel, simply because you are *understanding what you are doing as you do it*. Seeds—even good seeds—planted from either of the two side channels ultimately always end up giving us pain. Seeds planted from the middle channel always end up, eventually, creating a perfect world—for all of us. So *remember*," I finished.

We sat for a moment in that warm glow of the definite possibility of a perfect world. And then I broke the spell and said, "Captain, I think we'd better cover that second step in planting higher seeds at our next class. Otherwise we'll never get to the poses today."

He made a face, and I thought I heard a chuckle— whether from behind the wall or behind the door, I'm not quite sure.

37

Joy

Third Week of November

Before the first class with Busuku's little flock of eight boys, I pulled Ajit off to the side and told him *he* would be doing the teaching. He needed very powerful seeds to see his body change so much, and I seized the opportunity.

"Yes, Miss Friday," he said in that sunny gentle way he had. "I can tell them about the wonderful game with your breath during the silent sitting—where you take away bad things that happened to people and destroy those things inside you, and where you send everyone everything their heart desires. And then when it's time to do the poses, I will call you."

I shook my head gently. "No, Ajit. You don't understand. You will teach them *everything. Including* the poses."

He turned those lovely big brown eyes to me, and looked as if he were about to cry. "I mean, Miss Friday . . . I really am getting much better, you see, and I know it, and I . . . I thank you very much." And then he paused, struggling for the words. "But you . . . you see, I *can't even do* many of the poses myself yet."

"Nonsense," I blurted back, as Katrin would have. "Of course you can do them. You do all of them, every class we have together."

"Oh no," he said quietly. "No, no—it's not so, though you are so kind to say it, Miss Friday. I mean, I try—I always try to do the best I can—but my leg, you see . . . it changes everything else I try to do, and I know it. I know that with many poses what I do still isn't what the pose is *supposed* to look like."

I took his scarred cheek in my palm, and he let me, innocently—did he know it already looked better? "There's something you have to understand, Ajit. It's very simple and very true. A pose isn't *supposed* to look like *anything*. *Nobody* can do a pose so it *looks* perfect. A pose is *perfect* only when you are doing the very best you can—gazing steadily, breathing sweetly, and thinking of how it will help someone else. And I watch you every day, doing lots of these perfect poses. And that's the kind of poses I want our wonderful boys to learn."

He looked up at me with that instant brilliant faith of the young, and smiled, and nodded that yes, he would do as Teacher asked.

φ

"You'll be happy to know," I told the Captain, "that the second step to planting good seeds so they won't wear out is quite short and simple. Here the Master says only,

Use joy.

I.33c

Now we have to talk a little about this 'joy,' because it's not just regular joy. The Master mentions it in a famous list called the 'infinite thoughts,' and here it means something altogether special.

"So we go back to you helping the corporal do a yoga pose that will make him healthier; you as you preserve life, honor life, which is the opposite of harming others. And you are remembering to keep your mind on how everything going on at that very moment—you, the corporal, and the pose—are all three actually neutral or blank: they are no way at all from their own side. But rather they are what they are because of the way the seeds in your mind are making you see them; just like the green stick that can equally be a pen or a tasty treat, to two separate minds with very different seeds going off in them.

"And now on top of that you take the second step: you use what the Master calls 'joy.' Here 'joy' means wishing, at the moment that you help the corporal, that the help you are giving him could bring him a higher kind of goal. I mean, not just a body that is healthier for a while and then gets old and dies anyway. Instead you are wishing that this little good deed could eventually help him rid his own mind—and channels—of every single last negative emotion, forever. And then you make a wish that his channels could eventually become so pure and clear that it causes his body to become a body of living crystal light, and his mind to become perfect kindness and knowledge.

"Then you go one step more: you make your wish *infinite*. It *has* to be infinite if the seed you are planting is also to be infinite, and that's why this kind of joy is called an 'infinite' thought. Because at that moment, as you assist the corporal in an ordinary yoga pose, you must try to imagine that this small kindness you are doing will help turn *every single living creature* on *countless worlds* into this same perfect living crystal of kindness. And then in the instant that the imprint of your small act is planted in your consciousness, it is filled with good wishes for an infinite number of living creatures.

"This incredible change in the seed as it is planted in your mind makes it give a much different result as it begins to ripen. You see, the only way that every being alive now upon every planet there is can escape from death, and reach a pure body of light, is if they *can actually carry out* all the kinds of kindness we've been talking about. And to do this they need to understand *how* to do a true act of kindness— infinitely, and with an awareness of how seeds create things from neutral stuff. And no one could ever do this without carefully learning these ideas from a teacher who is already very familiar with them.

"And there comes a time, a very sacred moment in your life, when you realize that it is *you*—and you *alone*—who must decide to *be* this teacher, for countless living beings. It means being able to go to countless people on countless planets at the same time; it means knowing exactly what they need to learn, exactly when they need to learn it; and it means *knowing* yourself all there is to learn, because you have *finished* learning it, and because you yourself have already undergone the ultimate transformation.

"And so what I mean is—if you just *wish* that infinite numbers of living beings could be helped in an ultimate way through even just a few minutes of helping the corporal with his tummy—then higher seeds will be planted in your own mind. And when they ripen they will ripen in an ultimate way, in an infinite way: you *will* become a being of infinite light, helping infinite numbers of people on infinite planets reach this infinite ability as well: the ultimate form of happiness, the ultimate form of *joy*.

"And seeds planted with these wishes never wear out, you see. Every time a good seed ripens and brings you something good—say, a sound and healthy body—then you immediately turn around and use that healthy body to help *others* become healthy. And *that* puts the seed back into the ground of your mind, growing infinitely more powerful with each day, with each re-investment of what the seed has brought you. Over and over, taking the best seeds from this year's crop, planting them for next year's larger crop, onward into infinity, until you become this being of light who can act for others, infinitely, appearing at the side of anyone who needs you, in whatever form would best help them move towards this ultimate goal themselves."

The Captain was staring at me. And then he said, "Are you actually . . . suggesting . . . that we change that radically? I mean, not just overcome death—not just reach the ability to help the Sergeant and the corporal and . . . my lost wife and child—but actually become able to help an infinite number of others, all at the same time?"

"It is what each of us is meant to be," I said simply, "and deep inside, you know that."

38

Taking Not Thinking

Fourth Week of November

I opened the door to the Captain's office a week later, and suddenly there was a loud banging noise from outside. The Captain's eyes shot up with concern, and he flew past me, out to the porch. I raced after him, followed closely by the Sergeant.

We clustered around the source of the noise: the corporal, standing on top of a little stool, hammering nails into the old wooden poles of the roof over the front porch.

He suddenly caught sight of us, and said brightly, "Oh my! Time to start the Captain's class? I'm so sorry! Have to finish this up later!" And he leaped nimbly down to the porch, set the hammer on the stool, and slapped the dust from his hands.

"Corporal!" cried the Captain. "Corporal! What! What . . . *what* are you doing?"

The corporal looked confused. "Why, why . . . fixing the roof over the porch, sir! It's been half fallen down for . . . for as long as I can remember, sir!"

"Yes, yes, I know," replied the Captain hastily. "But . . . but what I mean is, *who told you* to fix the roof?"

"Why no one, sir," answered the corporal, but the Captain couldn't even hear it. He whirled around to the Sergeant.

"Sergeant, did you instruct the corporal here to fix the roof?"

"Wasn't me sir," said the Sergeant.

The Captain's eyes passed to me. "Not me!" I peeped.

"*No one* told me, sir," repeated the corporal, but still the words stopped short of the Captain's ears.

"Wasn't *me*," came a voice from the back.

"Shut up, Busuku," yelled the Sergeant, automatically, and then glanced at me and added, "Please," in a whisper.

And then we were all silent, and we just stared at the corporal together, dumbfounded, and he stared back in utter incomprehension and then finally said, "Going to need some more nails, Captain, sir."

φ

"Seeds!" said the Captain back at his desk, shaking his head in disbelief.

"Seeds!" I agreed in amazement, and then we got down to business.

"I think this will make the rest of the forms of self-control more fun," I said hopefully. "Because now we can imagine doing them with bigger things in mind."

The Captain hesitated a moment. "Miss Friday, I've been thinking about . . . about that idea of someone like me being able one day say to show up in three different houses . . . "

"Or three different *planets*," I reminded him.

"Er . . . yes, well—whatever. Anyway I need you to tell me a little bit more about how that works before . . . before I can really go about *wishing* for it, as I help the corporal, say . . . "

"I understand," I said. "And it's a fair request. But let's finish up the last three forms of self-control first, so you know *what* things are good seeds to turn into *higher* good seeds."

Then I paused for a moment. "But one more thing to add about never telling a lie," I said. "You need to know that here in the Master's *Short Book* it really covers three other very common things we do as well. The Master has only mentioned this one, speaking honestly, to stand for *all* the different ways we can plant good seeds as we speak. And of all these different ways, there are three crucial ones that you should know about.

"The first is to avoid ever speaking in a way that might split other people up—that might make them upset at each other. It could be two people who are friends, or who already have a problem. And it could even be that what you say to alienate one from the other is *true*. But we should never knowingly *try* to take people apart from one another: there is enough of that going on all the time, and it's so easy to fall into this just talking to people.

"If on the other hand we purposely try to encourage people to come together—if we emphasize to people the good things they can share with each other—then we automatically prevent seeds that would make us have trouble in all of our own relationships.

"Next here is to avoid ever saying something to someone else that would hurt their feelings: I mean, you could call it using harsh words. And you know that even the words

'Have a nice day' can be said in a way that hurts another's feelings . . . "

"In the same way that 'You are really a donkey!' can be said in a *friendly* way, I suppose," mused the Captain. "I mean among the three of us officers here, say," he added.

"Oh yes," I smiled. "That's right, and then they *aren't* harsh words.

"And then lastly there's perhaps the most difficult of all, which is avoiding useless talk. I mean, most of us like to talk all day long, whether there's anything important to say or not. And aside from wasting a lot of our time, we are likely to slip up and say a good number of negative things whenever we have a long rambling conversation with no particular purpose.

"And you know I'm not talking about talking to someone who's lonely, or to be friendly. Then we can usually control what we say. I'm talking about just talking for talking's sake. I mean, explore the beauty of silence, and get your friends to appreciate it too, and make it a goal with each other to try to be able to be together and enjoy each other's warmth and company even *without* having to talk, you see."

"I do see," replied the Captain, "and I do know what you mean. It's amazing how refreshing it can be to share silent moments with people you really enjoy. I can see how all of these would plant some wonderful seeds, say to live in a quiet, peaceful place; or to be exposed to beautiful music; or to be around friends who say sweet and heartfelt things all the time. I get it."

"Good," I said. "So let's go on. Now the Master says,

> *The third form of self-control*
> *Is never to steal from another.*
> II.30c

Now everybody knows what stealing is, and everybody knows that it's not a good thing to do, and most of us would say that we aren't in the habit of stealing things.

"But as usual, we have to go deeper. We have to be sensitive to anything that we ever do that could *amount* to stealing, even if we don't usually think of it that way. And then if we ever hope to get close to that idea of becoming a kind of angelic being who could help an infinite number of other people all at once, well then we have to go further and explore all the different ways we could *give* things to others, rather than *taking* things away from them.

"I mean, what I sometimes fantasize about," I said, gazing at the ceiling, "is a world where everyone already understands this stuff about things only being what the seeds in your mind make them to be. And then everyone is dying to be kind and helpful to each other, and so you have a new breed of burglar develop, say. I mean, they sneak into people's houses at night, and find their wallets, and *stuff* money into them, and then run away."

The Captain looked disturbed. "It would put us out of business," he said. And then suddenly he brightened up. "Or else, there could be, say, a new breed of *jail*, where we go and catch these new burglars and lock them up, so people can come and have classes with them every day. Why, it's exactly what we're already doing!" he said with pride.

"Er . . . right," I said, and went on.

"Now the point is that we want to become real experts at the art of non-stealing. Then it will plant some powerful seeds in us that change everything that's going on around us. The Master even goes so far as to say,

> *If you keep up this practice*
> *Of never stealing from anyone,*

Then there will come a time
When people just come to you
And offer you all the money you need.

II.37

And if you really think carefully about it, you see, he's exactly right. I mean, if you are very wise about planting your seeds properly—always being careful to respect others' things, always giving others whatever you can—then of course there comes a day when your own mind forces you to see whatever money you could ever need, and more, simply coming to you free. Because *all the money there is in the world*—every last little penny in the entire economy of our planet—is being created by the minds of those who own and use this money, as surely as the pen."

The Captain stopped and thought for a moment. "But there's a problem with that," he said uncertainly.

"What's that?" I said.

"I mean, suppose everyone in the world was very careful to respect everyone else's things, all of the time, and to be generous with what they already had themselves. According to you, then everyone would begin getting wealthy, everyone everywhere, at the same time."

"So?" I said.

"Well, where's it all going to come from?" he said slowly, and then actually winced when the voice boomed from behind the wall.

"Seeds, of course!"

And then, from behind the door, two more voices, one after the other: "From the same place that all the money there is *now* comes from anyway . . . " " . . . of *course!*"

The Captain got red, but smiled. And he looked up out of the window and mused, "Everyone, everywhere, could always have enough . . . the whole idea of there not being enough, the whole idea of how to capture or allocate or distribute wealth is . . . is simply . . . one big . . . " and then he yelled at the wall, before the wall could yell at him, ". . . one big *mistake,* of our *entire civilization,* for as long as it's been around!"

"*Bravo!*" returned the wall. I smiled and looked around. Surely at some point it was going to be less of a disruption to just have everyone come in together for class.

"Now a few points about how to respect others' things on the very subtle level you need to if you want to see your own world change. Just some food for thought; I'm sure you'll come up with others.

"It seems to me that most of us rarely outright *steal* something from another individual. I think rather we are more likely to get into common cultural situations that involve taking what is not ours, but perhaps not fully realizing it.

"I think first that when we deal with *public* property we get careless. I mean, just for a simple example, we could go into a public bathroom in a building in the city say, and leave behind a little mess that we would never leave in our own bathroom at home. And then someone will have to come and clean it up later on; and if you think about it, then we have stolen a little bit of the most precious thing a person has: not their money, but the short precious moments of their life."

"But what if they get *paid* to come in and clean up after people?" objected the Captain.

"Even worse," I said. "Remember we said it was a *public* building. And so ultimately whatever it costs to clean up the little messes that we make—even just what it costs to clean up the litter that people thoughtlessly toss on the street—this money is being *taken* from the pockets of *everyone* around us: from everyone who gives up part of their hard-earned pay in the form of taxes. What I mean to say is, we are often stealing therefore from everyone around us, without thinking.

"And taxes themselves—I mean, we should feel it an honor to help pay our fair share of the cost of things that we all use together: roads, bridges, systems for communication. But we are just selfish and want the money for ourselves, and so we try to cheat; and then whatever we don't pay must be extracted from everyone else, and again we are stealing from all those around us."

"Hogwash!" exclaimed the Captain. "There are so many bad and useless things that our taxes go towards!"

"Surely so," I agreed, "but in that case we should stand up, and speak out openly and honestly, to correct these wrongs—even go so far as to refuse to pay a wrong or harmful tax, if need be, and then suffer gladly whatever consequences there may be for us personally. But not by sneaking around like thieves, actually taking from everyone else.

"And it's the same when you work for someone; I mean, that's another very common form of stealing unaware. Someone hires you to work for so many hours a day, for so much money each hour, and most often you are very glad for the chance, at first. And then slowly you get lazy, or dissatisfied, and it becomes a game of doing as little work as you can during you appointed hours—talking with friends, drinking tea, avoiding extra tasks.

"And you see, the employer—he's not stupid. He will get the work done by taking extra time and effort from others who will or must give it. And then again you have failed to carry your fair share—what you have *promised* to carry by accepting the job in the first place—and again you are stealing, from others, their most precious life-time."

"But what about . . . what about if the employer is hard or unpleasant to you? What if they are unfair when it comes to respecting *your* needs, and *your* precious life-time?"

"Again, that's a *separate* issue," I pressed on. "From our side we must demonstrate integrity, and continue to work as we have first promised to work, until we choose to leave that job. And if unfair or improper demands are put on us—or upon anyone else around us, for that matter—then we must have the courage to stand up openly and work to change it, whatever the *apparent* consequences to ourselves. For remember: a good action cannot bring a bad result. Impossible."

The Captain took the very tiniest glance at one of the stacks of reports at his side, and then brought his eyes back to mine.

"And I think of one more way in which we can steal from others without being aware of it," I said. "It is when we steal from the others around us who do not have enough to eat, or to clothe or shelter themselves—and it is when we steal from our children, for generations to come—by using the resources around us selfishly and wastefully.

"Every time we use a thing we don't really need; every time we eat food far beyond what our bodies really require; every time we have extra—anything—when others have none, then we are stealing from the resources that all of us share now, and that people who come after us will need. And this surely plants a seed within us—constant seeds, countless seeds—that will deny us all that free and perfect wealth which the Master spoke of."

With that, the Captain sat up and openly gazed at the stacks of papers around him, chewing on his thumbnail nervously. And then finally he sighed and said, "We have to talk about something . . . "

"Next class," I replied, and again there was that same chuckle from somewhere outside the room, as I pulled him up for his poses.

39

Beginning the End of Old Bad Seeds

First Week of December

It was a satisfying time. Everybody was getting better—inside and out. I could often hear the Sergeant and the corporal engaged in animated discussions up in the side room, about things that they heard: both scraps through the Captain's door, and from their classes with the Captain himself. I could see that he had a real talent for teaching, and the results were certainly brightening up our little world.

Busuku's boys loved the yoga; they instantly learned to respect the idea of a perfect pose being any one which was done to the very best of one's honest ability, and in this no one could deny that the Sergeant's quiet boy was the unquestioned master. And so he too became a fine teacher, and I could see the powerful seeds from it literally changing his face and leg, day by day.

With Busuku himself though there was a problem one day.

The class with the boys was too big too fit in my cell, and so we would just open up the door with the crossbar that wasn't a crossbar and have some of the boys on one side of the bars and the rest on the other. And then once in a while Long-Life and I would get up to straighten a leg, or lick a hand for encouragement (I did the straightening).

And Busuku, well, he had this slightly imperious way about him, and—after all—they were *his* boys, and so he would stand up during class with his hands on the bars of his cell and yell out suggestions and corrections and cheers and jeers—as needed—to the boys that he could see. And then one day he told me that he could tell that the boys who needed his leadership the most were all moving inside my cell for class—where he couldn't see them. And I checked it for a few days and discovered that he was quite right, as usual.

And then Busuku said we really had to get him a crossbar like mine, you see—sawed in half—but I said that it really seemed to be up to the Sergeant you see, and so the scene was set for a confrontation.

The Sergeant was sitting in my cell for a moment after a class, with his son. The other boys had already gone—home? I often wondered where that was.

"Ravi! Oh Sergeant Ravi, sir!" called Busuku from the other side of my wall.

"Uh-oh," smiled the Sergeant softly. "He wants something."

"Sergeant, sir," began Busuku, and then it all poured out. "Ravi, my good fellow, now see here. First of all, I am the senior prisoner in this jail, and so I really should be able to ask for a simple privilege that—well, frankly—*other*, more *junior* prisoners of the jail already enjoy."

The Sergeant rolled his eyes. "I assume he means you *and* Long-Life," he said to me quietly, and Ajit looked up from scratching the little lion in his lap, and smiled.

"Secondly, and most importantly—and I must say that our yoga expert, Miss Friday herself, is in perfect agreement with me—it is of paramount importance that I be able to move around the entire outside room there, and even the neighboring cell, in order to impart my own not insubstantial fund of yoga knowledge to *my* boys during their classes here. As such, I require . . . "

"Busuku," sighed the Sergeant, "just say it."

"Ravi, you gotta get me a crossbar on my door like Miss Friday has."

The Sergeant's forehead wrinkled. "I don't know, Busuku. I mean we do need to keep up some appearance of incarceration here. I mean—what would the public think? And the Captain? And—goodness forbid—what if the Superintendent himself walked in?"

"Superintendent!" snorted Busuku. "Why he's nothing—I could take care of that myself, in a minute!"

"Sure, Busuku," said the Sergeant wearily.

"So I don't get the crossbar?" returned Busuku.

"Well, I'm not sure," said the Sergeant. "I'll have to think about it."

"I knew you'd say no."

"I *didn't* say no."

"I *knew* you'd say no, and I *knew* you wouldn't have the guts to say it too."

"I *don't* not have the guts, I just don't *want* to say no."

"Then you're saying no, then."

"No, I'm not!"

"There it is—you just did!"

"No I didn't."

"Again! Twice! How many nos is no no?"

"No! I mean, yes! I mean, Busuku, see here!"

"See here, no! I *knew* you'd say no! And I made a *plan* for when you said no! And you'll be sorry you said no!"

And then we heard some frantic scraping and tugging and then shortly afterwards a low groan.

"Busuku ... Busuku!" exclaimed the Sergeant with concern. "What are you doing?"

"You'll find out!" came a strained voice. "And you'll be *sorry!*" And then there was a low, heart-rending moan.

"Busuku!" cried the Sergeant, leaping up. "*What are you doing?*"

"I *told* you Ravi! See if you can sleep after this one! I'm over here doing an *Unsupported Headstand Pose*, and I'm going to stay this way until ... " there was another painful moan ". . . sorry—my head's getting all red, all puffed up like a watermelon already, you see — I'm going to stay this way *until my head explodes* or ... "

"Or what, Busuku?"

"Or until ... " another groan ". . . oh, the pain! Or until you agree to give me the crossbar ... Oh! Oh!"

I looked up at the Sergeant quickly. "Scrgeant sir ... he really shouldn't even *be* in that pose yet at all—I haven't gone over with him how to do anything close to that properly; he really could hurt himself."

Another groan, and then some popping sounds, like somebody sticking their finger in their mouth and popping their cheek.

The Sergeant rushed for the door and stopped dead just outside, staring heart-struck at the next cell.

Ajit and I scrambled to our feet. "Sergeant!" I cried.

And "Busuku!" the Sergeant cried. And we rushed out to see what the Sergeant saw: Busuku, sitting on the ground, facing my wall, his eyes closed in the middle of a deep groan, having just made another pop with—yes—his finger in his cheek.

"Busuku!" roared the Sergeant. "That's not a Headstand Pose at all!"

Busuku opened his eyes and looked up at us, and gulped.

"Er . . . er . . . right you are, Sergeant." Then he touched his finger to his head in thought. "It's rather . . . well, you see . . . the *preparatory position* for the Unsupported Headstand Pose, you see," he concluded reasonably.

Then he added, in a guilty voice, "Does this mean . . . I don't get the crossbar, Ravi?"

"No!" roared the Sergeant. And then, "I mean . . . yes!"

φ

Before I could say a word at our next class, the Captain held up his hand. "Wait," he said simply, and then turned and took a pile of papers off the stack closest to him.

"My reports . . . to the Superintendent," he said wryly. "All made up—all of them lies, to make us look good." He set his hand on top of the papers, with his head bent down, thinking.

"I mean, let me put it bluntly, Miss Friday. Anyone sitting and reading this part of the first and greatest book ever written about yoga must be thinking the same thing I'm thinking by now.

"I mean, if you really think over everything he's said so far—first, about things not really being themselves, from their own side. Second, how the way we personally see everything must then be coming from *our* side. Third, how seeds in our own mind force us to see what we do see. And fourth, how those seeds are planted every time we do, or say, or even think something good or bad towards others.

"And then when the Master starts going through his short list of the most powerful ways of planting both good and bad seeds, well, I mean, *anyone* who has grasped the different ideas in the *Short Book* up to here—anyone who really cares about what's going to happen to them, including me—well, by now, you've *got* to be thinking about all the seeds you've *already* planted in your life: about mistakes you've made, about the mistakes that we've all made, which must have hurt other people—some very seriously.

"And me, personally, thinking about what happened with the Sergeant, and then his boy; or thinking about so much of the work I've done since I've sat in this office—so many lies, so much stealing really from so many others—I mean, I want to know if you'd be willing to say something today about how we can stop or remove the bad seeds that we *know* we already have in our mind, waiting to go off. It seems doubly important to me if—as we said before—these seeds are constantly gathering power, doubling and tripling constantly every single day that passes until they finally ripen and make us see something really painful. Because if there's no way to stop the ones we already have, then I can't see a lot of hope for just normal people, like myself."

I nodded; it was time. "I think you're right," I said. "I think we should cover this now; and then later we'll go on with the last two forms of self-control."

"Thank you, Miss Friday," said the Captain, with a sound of relief that made me realize he really understood how important this part was, if we ever hoped for anything good to happen in our lives.

"Now the Master begins this point by saying,

> *When the images*
> *Start to hurt you,*
> *Sit down and work*
> *On the antidote.*

II.33

The 'images' he's talking about are all the painful things that bad seeds will make you see. These things will hurt you, unless you can stop them first. I mean, you can either stop a bad thing before it happens, or you can stop *the rest*—or the *future*—of a bad thing that is already happening; something like your bad back, if you can get at the bad seeds already planted in your mind. And this is what the Master calls the 'antidote': a very clear series of concrete steps found throughout the ancient books; steps that you can sit down and work on, to stop bad seeds before they go off.

"Now here are the steps you have to go through; there are four, and the Master begins the first one by saying,

The images—
People who hurt me or the like—
Come from what I did myself;
Or got others to do for me;
Or what I was glad to hear
Others had done.

II.34A

The point is that the first step in going into your own mind and destroying bad seeds that you know are there is to go back to the basics: go over what you have planted by mistake, and how you planted it. And that means, first of all, really recognizing *that* you did something to plant a seed. Here before anything else the Master wants to remind us that there are three ways of planting a seed, either good or bad.

"The first way, obviously, is just by doing or saying or even just thinking something negative, and *watching* ourselves as we do it—which, as you know, is what *plants* the seed in our minds.

"But the Master also wants us to know that whenever we get someone *else* to do something harmful for us, then the seed is planted in *us* all the same. So it doesn't matter who else does the dirty work, if you're behind it."

The Captain lifted a finger. "Does that mean that the person we get to do the bad thing for us *doesn't* get a seed?"

"No," I replied. "They do too—you both do. And so you get the *extra* seed of making *them* get a seed that will hurt *them*."

"Oh," he said glumly, his mind off again on past bad seeds he hadn't even known about.

"And then lastly there are all the negative seeds that we plant just by being glad about negative things that we've heard other people have done, even if we didn't ask them to personally. These seeds are not as strong as the ones we plant when we do something ourselves, but they add up quickly since we are so often glad say that someone we don't like has gotten hurt, even if we are too 'civilized' to have hurt them ourselves."

The Captain paused again to calculate these seeds, and shook his head in exasperation. "Better get to the seed-destruction part fast!" he wheezed.

"But this *is* the seed-destruction part, at least the first step of it. You have to stop and think carefully about how the seeds work, in order to get at them before they ripen into people who come to hurt you, or anything else of the like: images, like a bad back, that ripen from the seeds to deliver us our pain.

"Remember again that we can also destroy seeds that have *already* ripened into problems; that is, we can stop them from *continuing*, no matter how old the problem might be—even one that you've had as far back as your birth. In cases like this the seed is too old to remember planting it; so we have to stop and think about what it *probably* was, given our current problem. If it's a very old health problem, for example, we can assume that the seed was planted by hurting someone else, even if we don't remember doing it. And then we work from there."

"Got it," he said, and I could see him taking mental notes furiously.

"The Master continues then on the first step by saying,

And what came before them
Was either craving, or hating,
Or dark ignorance.

II.34B

You see, whenever we do something negative, one of three bad thoughts has to come before. The Master has covered them earlier, when he went through the various negative thoughts . . . " I paused for him.

"Ah yes," said the Captain, almost immediately. "These must be our old friends: liking things stupidly, disliking things stupidly, and then misunderstanding them in the first place, in all its different flavors."

"Exactly," I said. "And these three are also known as the 'three poisons,' because they poison our hearts and make us then do things that would hurt people . . . "

". . . And plant seeds to hurt ourselves," he added.

"Let's check," I said. "Examples?"

The Captain didn't have to think long. "The corporal comes in this morning and asks me the dumbest question . . . "

"Which was?"

"I mean, he wants to know if we can take that old abandoned cow that ate my . . . pen, and keep it in back, and take care of it."

"That's stupid?"

"Well yes," said the Captain defensively. "There's no room for a cow behind the jail. Completely out of the question."

"I see."

"Yes, and well, so . . . when he asks this stupid question I am faced immediately with a choice. One, I can see him as being stupid from his own side—which is as completely impossible as a pen that was a pen from its own side, and therefore also a fully functional pen even to the same ridiculous cow in question.

"Two, I can see him as being stupid because *I* was, say, purposely unpleasant to someone else in the past—say, said something that hurt their feelings.

"Now if I choose the first option and see him as annoying from his *own* side . . . "

"Which is what the Master calls 'dark ignorance' here," I added.

"Yes . . . then, well—since it's not *my* fault then, you see, then I can start *disliking* him *stupidly*."

"What the Master calls 'hating' here," I added again.

"And then I'm well on my way to, to well calling him a nincompoop, and seeing him get hurt and almost start to cry and run out the door."

"Oh no, really?" I asked.

"Er, why . . . yes," said the Captain, a little sadly. "But anyway, then I've just planted a seed in my *own* mind to see someone say something bad to *me*, again — which is what started the whole thing in the first place. And so the vicious Circle is set in motion one more time."

307

"And what about an example for what the Master calls here 'craving'?" I asked.

"That's pretty easy," said the Captain. "It's why I wanted to talk about getting rid of old bad seeds in the first place. Say I am like anyone working for someone else, and I want my boss to be happy with me. In my case, that would be the Superintendent.

"And it's not *wrong* to want your boss to be happy," he continued. "It's a good thing, in fact. But suppose you want this thing the wrong way: you like it *stupidly*, or *crave* it in a way that comes from *misunderstanding* it—from this dark kind of ignorance.

"Which is to say, you forget that if you see the Superintendent walk in and compliment you on a job well done, it's got to be happening because of good seeds you planted before, when you yourself spoke with honesty and encouragement to someone else.

"And if you forget *that*, then, you might fall into that old most stupid way of viewing the world around you: you might be tempted to do that most stupid of all things and try to force a *good* result to happen (which is the boss giving you a compliment) by doing something *bad* to cause it (say, by writing false reports)."

"Or even just *exaggerated* reports," I added.

"Oh no! Really? I mean . . . just a little exaggeration? Surely that's not a problem!"

"It's a kind of lying," I said bluntly. "The pictures don't match. We went through that already."

"Then what you're basically saying is . . . is that we all have to live like saints!" he objected.

"Saints, or better . . . ," I mused. "I'll be honest with you Captain. It takes a tremendous amount of good seeds—and it takes removing a tremendous amount of old bad seeds—if you want to have any hope of actually seeing you and your world change into the most beautiful living light of all. You have to give it your whole heart; your whole effort. And countless others are depending on you, depending on each of us, to do it. Yes, we do have to be good—very good, and we have to know *why* we are, and *how* to do it.

"And that brings us to the end of the first step in destroying old bad seeds; I think we'll cover this and then do the rest at our next session. Here the Master says,

> *They are of lesser, or medium,*
> *Or greater power.*
>
> II.34c

I mean, you have to know what makes one seed more powerful than another; because when you get into the business of destroying old bad seeds, you have to go after the most powerful ones first.

"The first consideration here is the relative seriousness of the act. I mean—under normal circumstances—it's much more serious to kill someone for example than to lie to them. That point's pretty obvious. What you might not guess is that the most serious mistake of all is simply to hold or to spread a view of the world which is mistaken . . . " I waited to see if the Captain would pick it up.

"I can guess what you mean by that," he said. "I mean, suppose it really is true that if you can learn to do even small good deeds constantly, but with infinite hopes of benefit for infinite beings as you do so—then you can actually become . . . like an angel, who can go anywhere and help anyone.

"And suppose instead you thought that say your own body comes from its own side: I mean, suppose your view of things said that they had to be the way they seem to be now, because they come from themselves.

"And then suppose you influenced other people to think that way too, perhaps without even thinking much about it. Well I guess then that you would have deprived them of something even more precious than whatever mortal life they have left to them anyway. And so a simple way of viewing things can kill more people than any physical action at all," he concluded.

"I'm afraid so," I agreed. "And that would be the most powerful bad seed of all, you see, and the first one we'd want to go after." He nodded and added it to his mental notes.

"Now seeds are also more powerful if what we do is directed towards a more potent object. I mean, all life is precious—equally precious. But if we were to say kill a physician who was himself already engaged in saving the lives of many sick people, it would plant a much more powerful seed than killing someone who wasn't so engaged. And so we'd want to make sure to try to stop any seed we had ever created by hurting someone who was especially kind or helpful, you see.

"Doing something negative with very strong emotions can also make a seed much more powerful. It's one thing to harm another person out of a strong feeling of hatred; it's another thing to hurt them almost by accident. And here too we have to mention *intention*, which is perhaps the biggest factor of all. A big mistake done towards someone can make a much smaller seed if our intention was neutral, or even good: say when a child kills an animal not because of any kind of hatred, but only to please a parent who doesn't know any better themselves.

"You see, if it is the very fact of how we *see* ourselves do an action that plants a bad or a good seed in our minds, then *intention*—which is almost our own awareness of ourselves as we act—is crucial, the most crucial factor of all."

"Then do we plant a bad seed say if we kill a person in an accident, on the road?"

"You do," I said, "simply because the deed was *done*. But the seed is infinitely less than if you'd done it intentionally— on purpose."

"Seems to work a lot like a normal court of law," said the Captain.

"It does," I said, "for it's mostly only common sense. And except of course that justice is *always* done impartially: the rules which govern seeds are as cold and unforgiving as something like the law of gravity—if you step off the roof of a building, you're going to fall. And so you have to work within these rules to stop the seeds before they have a chance to flower.

"A few more points here, and then we'll get on with the poses. A seed is obviously more powerful if the negative thing you've done to plant it was something you'd *planned* to do, carefully: it's like pre-meditation in a crime. And a seed is obviously *less* powerful if you *try* to hurt someone but fail to do so.

"There's an element of recognition too: if you kill the town doctor but you had no idea he *was* the town doctor, then the seed is not as strong. And finally—and this is perhaps most important of all in *removing* old bad seeds—a lot of how strongly a seed is planted depends upon whether you decide to *own* it afterwards. That is to say, a seed's power is increased substantially if—after you hurt another person—you say to yourself, 'Good! I did it! He's been hurt, and I'm glad of it.'

"If on the other hand we succeed in hurting someone but then afterwards we step back and feel very sorry that we've hurt them, then seeds are planted to stop that very seed."

40

Old Debts Cancelled

The improvement in Mata Ji's gnarled fingers was amazing; I often felt that she had even more faith in the yoga and the yoga ideas I was teaching her than I did myself, and the results told the story. Her hands already felt so well that sometimes she would pick up a ball of yarn that I was using for a rug and twist the threads wistfully with her fingers, in a way that told me she had once weaved things herself, and missed it, and wanted to try again.

I was taking her out to the porch after class one day—and it was a lovely porch now, all straight and clean and freshly painted, all by the corporal, and all on his own. He himself burst out of the side room just then, with the Sergeant in tow; they nearly ran us over, rushed to the Captain's door, and knocked and threw the door open in a single motion.

"Captain sir!" exclaimed the corporal, and Mata Ji and I went to peek in, and see what all the excitement was about.

The corporal stood at the side of the Captain's desk and set a huge old dusty sheet of paper down on it.

"There it is, sir!" he announced.

"There's *what*, corporal?" asked the Captain, annoyed and already neglecting to ask who had planted the seeds for this latest irritating image of his subordinate. Ah well, I thought. It takes time, and practice.

"Yes, there it is!" repeated the corporal. "*Isn't it*, Sergeant sir?"

The Sergeant nodded hastily as the Captain repeated, "There's *what*, corporal? Sergeant . . . it's, I mean . . . there's . . . *what is this paper*?"

"Decree . . . ," began the Sergeant.

"Royal decree," burst in the corporal. "Royal decree granting the land that this jail stands on. And so we *can* keep the cow, and take care of her!"

"Wait a minute," said the Captain. "Sergeant, corporal, sit down here. Take it easy. What does the King have to do with a cow?"

"It's quite clear," rushed on the corporal, sitting and leaning over the desk and pointing to a section on the paper. "You see, the land we were granted for the jail — it goes back *hundreds of yards*, all the way to the stream beyond the trees out back.

"And that means we not only have plenty of land to keep all the animals . . ."

"What *animals*?" cried the Captain. "I thought we were talking about a cow. *One* cow."

The corporal looked up in the Captain's face with wounded disbelief. "Why, she's not just a *cow*, sir! She's a *mother*! She has a baby! We can't take her in and just tell her calf to go away! Why, she's been through that already! Probably got dumped out on the road one day when she couldn't pump out enough milk to pay for her feed! We can't put her through another trauma like that!"

The Captain's hand went by instinct back to his old bad back that wasn't bad any more, and then settled on his forehead instead.

"Corporal, I mean really. This is a *jail*, for goodness' sake, not a *zoo!* If you want to, you can just set out a bucket of leftovers or what-not for her on the porch every day, and leave it at that."

The corporal looked scandalized. "Sir! That would seriously detract from the tidy beauty of our newly refurbished porch! And don't forget that the Master himself says,

> The first commitment
> Is to cleanliness!"

The corporal looked over to the Sergeant for support. "That's what the book says," the Sergeant concurred.

"Moreover, Mrs. Cow would be very likely to damage the garden if she were allowed to come in the front gate whenever she pleased!" pointed out the corporal, supreme with logic.

"*What* garden?" asked the Captain, clutching his forehead in pain now.

"The *flower* garden out front!" explained the corporal patiently, as if the Captain had gone mad, or senile.

"But we don't *have* a flower garden out front," groaned the Captain. "Nor do we have a front *gate*," he wheezed.

"Got you there," said the Sergeant, pointing out the door. We all turned and saw a new and pretty little yellow gate, leaning up against the far wall.

"And the flowers—they're almost *all* planted already," continued the corporal excitedly. "And they're *not* the kind of seeds you'd want to stop before they ripened, sir! Why the Master says . . . "

"Spare me the Master," moaned the Captain. "I get enough of that from Miss Friday. Ravi, Sergeant . . . you, you figure it out with him; make sure he doesn't go overboard. Now leave me alone before I plant some really bad new seeds with my stick over there . . . "

φ

"So the first step in getting rid of your old bad seeds," I began at our next class, "is simply to go over what you did to plant them, reviewing everything you know about how they work.

"And then naturally, if you really grasp how your life in the coming months and years will be ruled by these seeds, you will start to wish you had never planted them."

"We should feel guilty about them, I guess," said the Captain.

I made a little face and thought about it. "I don't think 'guilty' is the right idea, Captain. In fact I don't think the ancient books even have a word for feeling 'guilty.' I mean, suppose you walk into your friend's house on a really hot day and you see a cup full of something that looks like juice on the table. And you know he wouldn't mind, and you just drink it all down in one big thirsty gulp. And then your friend rushes in with a loud cry and tells you you've just drunk a cup full of a very strong cleaner which happens to be highly poisonous. I mean, would you—at that very moment—feel *guilty?*"

The Captain laughed. "Guilty? No. Stupid? Yes. I'd mostly feel like finding out right fast how to get it back out of me. And at any rate I'd feel sorry I drank it, and I'd definitely resolve never to drink cups of unknown stuff at my friend's house ever again, should I live so long."

"That's the spirit," I said. "You see, it's not beating yourself up—it's thinking very clearly about the danger you've put yourself in, and doing something quickly to fix it. Guilt is useless, but regret spurs us on to take action to fix things. And the Master advises us next to think to ourselves like this:

> *Say to yourself then,*
> *"Who knows what pain*
> *I have planted for myself?*
> *The results could be countless."*
> *Sit and work out*
> *The antidote.*
>
> II.34D

And with this he covers the second step—which is just an honest and well-informed regret about the old bad seeds that you planted before you knew about seeds. It could also be thinking about *new* bad seeds you've planted *after* you knew better—but you just couldn't control yourself. Which is a very common situation that all of us who start out on the path of yoga find ourselves in frequently, as we are just beginning to put our new understanding into practice.

"This kind of intelligent regret—where you really understand the massive repercussions upon your mind and your reality of even just a small negative action towards another person—*feels* pretty bad but has one most wonderful result of its own: a lot like how you feel at your friend's house after the poison. I mean, you think to yourself—very, very clearly—'I will *never* do that again!'

"And if you want to know the *one thing* you can do to destroy an old bad seed from some serious mistake you may have made earlier in your life—this is *it*. *This* is what the

Master is talking about when he *repeats* 'sit down and work out the antidote,' and it's also the third step. Because the one thing that can really destroy the seeds of a past mistake is to make a definite decision that we will not *repeat* that mistake.

"If we have for example lied to our employer over a long period of time, and we know we have those seeds to face, then we can actually *destroy* those *particular* seeds by deciding, very consciously, that we will *not* lie that way again. And we dedicate this new power purposely to stopping those old seeds. But then of course we must actually *stick to* our decision, for it to work."

"Ah, now that really makes sense," said the Captain. And then he added, "Although it would be nice if there were an *easier* way of stopping the consequences of old bad things we've done—I mean, *really* not doing them *again* is undoubtedly a lot more difficult than it sounds."

"Well, there *is* no easier way," I said bluntly, "and that's just the way it is. I guess we should just be very happy that there *is* a way at all." Goodness, that *really* sounded like Katrin.

We sat for a moment and then I added, "One more thing though about resolving not to *repeat* a mistake, and *sending* that power consciously to stop an old bad seed."

"What's that?" asked the Captain.

"Well, there are some mistakes we make that are pretty easy to decide we will never do again: say a kind of killing, for example, once we have learned that it's wrong. But there are other mistakes we make that it would frankly be difficult to promise we will never repeat: say, getting mad at your boss, and yelling at him or her. And so the Masters of old, they used to say that—in order to avoid piling a new lie on top of our original mistake—we should in cases like this just make a commitment to avoid the same mistake again for a specific period: for a length of time that you can actually commit to. Say, promising not to yell at the boss again for a week, and then trying very hard to watch yourself for that long."

"That makes sense," said the Captain, and I could almost see him make another note on a list in his mind.

"Fourth step," I said, "and then you know all you need to know about stopping your old bad seeds before they go off in your mind. This is thinking of a concrete action that you could undertake which would be the *opposite* of what you did, just to show how much you regret it: something very tangible to 'make up' for the mistake."

"You mean, say, that I could call in the corporal and apologize for being rough on him?"

"That's one thing," I nodded, "and certainly *telling* someone—either the same person, or anyone else whom you really respect—goes a long way towards stopping the seed. But what we're talking about here doesn't necessarily have to be done with the person that you hurt.

"If say earlier in your life you had been involved in some business dealings that weren't very honest, and cost other people money, then as this sort of make-up activity you could work for some time at feeding hungry people. If you had been involved in a killing, you could dedicate some time to working as a volunteer in a hospital. But the most powerful 'make-up' of all is simply to set aside some time to sit quietly and go over in your mind how seeds draw pictures in our mind, and turn neutral objects into the very world around us."

"Just thinking about the pen and the cow?" asked the Captain, almost incredulous.

"Exactly so," I said. "That's what *really* kills old bad
seeds, and makes them *stay* dead. The Master even goes so
far to say,

> Contemplation on this point
> Destroys the storehouse of seeds.
> IV.6

And why do you guess that's so?" I asked.

The Captain thought for a moment, and then smiled
hugely. "Let's say you've been yelling at someone regularly.
And to make up for that, you decide to sit down and practice
thinking about how, say, a young man with a tummy is just
sort of a neutral collection of shapes and sounds.

"Now if *I* happen to experience those shapes and sounds
as an extraordinarily irritating junior officer, then it can *only*
be because I have been *just as irritating* to someone *else* in
the past—which planted seeds in my mind that are going
off now and making my mind see the shapes and sounds
as a pest.

"The point," he said then, "is that the more you sit down
and think about seeds, to make up for a mistake you've
made, then the less likely you are to *repeat* that mistake. And
not repeating our mistakes also just happens to be the third
step—the one that does the most towards destroying old
bad seeds."

"*Perfect!*" I smiled. "Perfect." And he sat for a moment
basking in the praise.

Then he asked, "Do you really think I can get rid of *all*
of them?" Because we both knew that some of his old seeds
were very serious.

"*Can*, and *must*," I affirmed. "For the very big seeds
you'll want to repeat the steps again and again, over say a

number of months. But then they will be gone, and you will feel it, a kind of lightness. And then you must know they are gone, and take joy in it, and never look back again. The Master says,

> *You will never have to pay*
> *Those old debts back;*
> *Not a single one.*

IV.29A"

41

The Spirit's Breath

Third Week of December

"Now the Master says that

> *Sexual purity*
> *Is the fourth form*
> *Of self-control.*

II.30D

In the ancient books, the expression that the Master uses here, 'sexual purity,' always refers to chastity, in the sense of refraining from every type of sexual activity. And the Master mentions it because his book was primarily intended in his own time for people who had already made that commitment.

"But he places this form of self-control in a position within the standard list where we know it also refers to the most common form of serious sexual misconduct, which is committing adultery with the sworn husband or wife of another person. And this is certainly one of the most harmful things we can do to someone else: a source of terrible pain and tragedy for many families."

We stopped and thought for a moment. "I think we have to talk about this one a little deeper," I said, "because there are so many strong emotions, and feelings of guilt, and questions that come up about sex in general. I think first we have to talk about why that's so, and then we can step back and clarify exactly where and how sexual activity could be right or wrong.

"People are deeply attracted to sex; it is an incredibly strong drive in almost everyone. And there's a reason for this, which goes back to those subtle channels and winds in the body that we spoke about before.

"You see—as we said—we have these winds inside us from the first moments of life within the womb. And by nature they are blocked—bottled up—because of areas where the two side channels wrap around the middle channel. Our very body forms around the pattern determined by these choke-points.

"Whenever we have those different negative thoughts—misunderstanding where the things around us really come from, and then liking or disliking things in an ignorant way because of this misunderstanding—then the subtle winds within us flow more powerfully in the two side channels. They then choke the middle channel even more strongly, and this is ultimately responsible for the fact that we grow older, and even for death itself.

"Now in the normal course of our lives, the middle channel stays choked almost completely, almost all the time. A strong thought, and therefore the wind upon which it rides, travel freely within the middle channel only on very rare occasions.

"One such occasion happens to occur during the process of dying itself, as the side channels dissolve, releasing their hold. But there are other moments too: moments of extreme compassion, incredibly fierce moments of love. In such a moment, anyone at all—even if they have no knowledge at all of the very existence of the channels and the knots—can suddenly feel what it's like for a major knot to loosen briefly, and a flash of pure inner wind to burst through the choke-point.

"A fierce emotion of love happens to trigger this momentary breakthrough at the knot located right behind the heart, which is why for centuries the heart has been associated with feelings of love, and compassion.

"And you must know that, whether they consciously understand anything at all about the channels and the knots, every person alive has a deep craving for that incredible feeling of the inner winds of life cracking through a knot, even briefly. When any amount of wind at all passes through the middle channel like this, even for a minute or two, it's as if our deeper body—our spirit itself—has been allowed to take a deep breath after years and years without any breath at all.

"Deep inside too every living person senses that—if this breath were allowed to go on, freely—then their entire being could change. For this is exactly how it happens that we make our transformation into a being of pure light. This is how we become a pure being who can appear on countless worlds to help countless people, all in the same moment.

"And this is our destiny, you see—it is what we all *will* become, and deep inside us we all know that, and crave desperately for that final moment.

"And you see, there is another moment in the life of any person, whether they know anything about channels or not, when a brief burst of wind, the spirit's breath, flies up the middle channel. And this is during the few peak moments of the sexual experience.

"And so, you see, this gives you some feeling of why the sexual drive is so powerful; why this craving too is so deep in people. It is so strong you see that it can blind a person for weeks or years to the repercussions of whatever actions they are driven to do to fill this urge. And so you will see normal people expend huge amounts of effort, spend sizeable portions of their wealth, and do things that hurt quite a few others, in order to fulfill the drive for sex.

"And it's not that sex itself is in any way wrong; the Master is not saying that it is. In the ancient books, sex between consenting persons who have reached what is considered a normal age of responsibility is fine, so long as they have no other commitments. But it is very wrong and destructive to have sex with a person who is sworn by marriage to another person, unless that bond has already been dissolved by a formal, mutual agreement.

"And the seeds that you plant by doing such harm to another person's spouse are very strong. They can prevent you for the rest of your life from having any happy experiences at all with those of the opposite sex: it is one of the main causes for the many sad and frustrated people who cannot find a suitable partner in life."

The Captain nodded, and thought for a moment. "It makes sense," he said, "as usual. And of course it helps explain why the same forms of self-control pop up in the teachings of great beings all over the world, and all through history." Then he thought some more.

"By what you just said," he mused, "do you mean to imply that—if we were able to keep sizeable amounts of wind flowing through the middle channel on a regular basis—we would feel like, I mean . . . like those few moments, with someone of the opposite sex . . . but *all the time?*"

"That's exactly right," I said. "And that's why people who are getting close to that point, you see—they move beyond sex altogether. They know that the sexual act can crack open the middle channel, but only for a few moments—and then it shuts back up again like a clam, and we feel worse than before. And they know that there are other ways of forcing this channel open, very briefly; I mean, certain kinds of drugs, certain herbs, have this power too, and with them we can sometimes glimpse for a few minutes what our ultimate future will be like.

"But people like this also know that these are not ways of *keeping* the middle channel open, you see; it takes a tremendous amount of time and thought and trouble to enjoy one of these experiences even for a few moments, and then you're always back to zero—or worse, if you've hurt someone or collected some bad seeds to get the experience.

"So these people have decided to dedicate all their time and effort to reaching the real method of keeping this middle channel open. Working at it from the outside, with the poses and the breathing exercises. Working at it from the inside, sitting silently and practicing infinite thoughts of kindness. *Doing* good for others, and destroying the seeds from past mistakes. Purposely creating the future garden: cultivating the seeds that would make you see the middle channel open wide, open forever, and a new body form around that.

"And on a practical level," I put on my Katrin voice, "that means, Captain, sticking to the Fortress Principle: don't even get *close* to a situation where you could damage a marriage. Here's an easy rule of thumb. Any time you are around anyone of the opposite sex who is married, say, even just a woman who comes to deliver a jug of water—" the Captain's eye twitched the slightest bit "—then never say anything to them that you wouldn't if their husband were standing right there next to them."

He looked out the window, and then slowly smiled. "All I was hoping for was a nice exercise program to fix my back. Now you're trying to turn me into light . . . " He paused.

Then he turned and said, "Let's do it!"

φ

The Sergeant came in out of the rain one day that week dragging a boy by the arm. I recognized him as Young Warrior, the first of Busuku's boys I'd ever met, outside on the path. He was wet and cold and shaking in his tattered shirt and shorts.

"Busuku!" roared the Sergeant. "Out here, now!"

"The . . . the crossbar, Ravi," I heard Busuku's voice, but I could tell it was no joke.

The Sergeant pulled off the bar, tossed it on the floor, and dragged Busuku out by the collar.

"Corporal!" he yelled. "Front and center!" The corporal walked sleepily out of the front room.

"Miss Friday! If you will!" called the Sergeant then, and he herded us all into the Captain's room.

The Sergeant pushed us all to the floor around the desk, and stood where he was before the flabbergasted Captain, pointing his finger down in Busuku's face.

"How *could* you?" he bellowed.

"Could . . . what . . . Ravi . . . sir?" blustered Busuku.

"*Look* at this boy!" glowered the Sergeant. "Half dead from the cold, and the rain! Found him and a bunch of the rest of them, all huddled under a big tree! Told me *that* was their *house!* Told me *that* was where they *lived!* I . . . I can't believe it! Busuku! How could you?"

Busuku let out one loud "Ah!" and then sat and thought for a moment; finally he nodded and pulled himself up tall. "See, here, Sergeant. And you too, Captain," and this time it was Busuku pointing his beefy finger.

"First of all, you can't keep me locked up all the time and still expect me to be stea. . . I mean, *providing* for my boys.

"Secondly, even when I was on the outside and times were good, I couldn't afford to keep a place for us. I mean, *I* was sleeping out under that tree with them too.

"And lastly, I never got any help from anyone. I mean, abandoned children wandering around town like the corporal's pet cow and calf and pig . . . "

"And *pig?*" interjected the Captain with concern. The Sergeant and the corporal hastily looked down.

"And so . . . I mean . . . *what else could I do?* What else would *you* do?" cried Busuku, glaring around the circle at each of us.

All was silent for a moment, and then the Sergeant said, "Well what's past is past. I'm talking about here and now. And I absolutely *refuse* to allow young people who attend our school . . . "

"Ravi," sighed the Captain. "This is not a school. It's a *jail*."

"Who attend our school jail . . . ," the Sergeant corrected himself.

Busuku shook his head. "It's not a school jail either. That doesn't sound so good."

"Jail school?" tried the corporal.

"Jail," repeated the Captain.

"School," I sneaked in.

"Anyway," continued the Sergeant righteously. "We absolutely refuse to allow our young people here to sleep out under a tree. Am I right?" He looked around at all the rest of us—everyone except the Captain—and we all nodded enthusiastically, perhaps influenced by some vague memory of his stick.

"But where are we going to put them?" asked the corporal.

The Sergeant stared at the ground, thinking furiously. "My house is full. You and your mother's is just a tiny thing. The Captain . . . " And here the Captain looked a little panicky.

"Sergeant," said the corporal quickly. "You know, it's better just to put them here."

The Sergeant's eyes brightened up. "Of course!"

"Cell wouldn't do," said the corporal.

"Records room—we'll clear it out; I mean, just temporarily," said the Sergeant.

"Oh right! And then expand the whole southern wall of the jail!"—the corporal.

"Certainly room there, according to the decree"—Sergeant.

"Share the structural wall?"—corporal.

"Exactly, break doors through after construction"—Sergeant.

"Water?"—corporal.

"Pipe it in by bamboo, from the back stream; decree stipulates right-of-way"—Sergeant.

Captain: staring from face to face, lost.

"Sanitation?"—corporal.

"Time to go underground"—Sergeant.

"Eight-inch baked brick?"—corporal.

"Best for a quick job"—Sergeant.

"Great, that's it. Everything's settled then. We can start tomorrow"—corporal.

"Captain sir; we've got your okay on that, right?" rushed the Sergeant.

The Captain stared at the other two in a complete daze, and nodded without knowing he was nodding.

The rest of us basked for several quiet moments in the glow of grand expectations for helping others. And then Busuku suddenly frowned, and cleared his throat, and looked over in my direction and said, "Er . . . may I ask, who's going to *pay* for all this?"

I shrugged and looked at the corporal.

He shrugged and glanced to the Sergeant.

He shrugged and turned towards the Captain, eyes pleading.

And the Captain came slowly out of his daze, and gazed slowly at our faces, and then at the stacks of papers all round. And then he said sadly, "Men, Miss Friday, Busuku—there's something I've been meaning to tell you. I mean . . . to be quite frank . . . I've made a decision, a personal decision, that I really can't go on any longer writing false reports of our accomplishments to the Superintendent."

There was a sudden little burst of applause from all the rest of us, before we'd even thought to do it. The Captain looked up with a broad smile, and wiped a little tear from his eye.

"Why . . . why thank you, I . . . I had no idea . . . that you would understand." And then he choked with emotion, and was quiet for a moment.

"And so," he continued then, "I must say that the three of us will need to actually . . . you see . . . get out more often, you see, and . . . actually . . . patrol around, you see, and . . . and help people who need us." Another burst of applause. The Captain reddened and smiled like a new bride.

"Right," he went on, "and thank you . . . thank you all again. But I'm afraid, you see, that this means that . . . well, at least for a while, we may not . . . we may not get nearly as much financial support as we used to. We'll all have to buckle down and tighten up our belts, for a while at least—until the new seeds kick in," he said confidently, glancing over at me. I gave him a big smile of encouragement for his courage.

"And that also means," he added slowly, "that I have absolutely no idea where we're going to find the money to build this addition onto our jail or school, for the children." And with that he sighed heavily, and sat back with a glum look.

Again, silence; all around, for some very long minutes. And then the corporal sat up and said firmly, "I'll take care of it."

42

Seeds of Thought

Fourth Week of December

After her class that next week, Mata Ji touched my hand warmly, then reached into a little cloth shoulder bag she always carried. She pulled out a small cloth bundle tied with a beautiful white ribbon made from the fibers of some local plant. "For you, my teacher," she smiled, and gestured at me to open it.

I did, and inside there was a small square seat carpet, woven into fantastic designs of great golden tigers. I felt a sudden pang in my heart, thinking of my mother and the Indian patterns of her own rugs; wondering if she were well, far off over the mountains to the north.

"It's so lovely," I said softly, and hugged her.

"For your silent sitting ... I made it myself," she whispered in my ear. And then she pulled away gently and held up her hands, waving her fingers like fronds of a palm tree.

"Oh *wonderful!*" I said, and we hugged again, for a long while.

Mata Ji held me by the shoulders then like a daughter and said, "Which brings me to a favor I'd like to ask of you."

I nodded quickly. "Of course; anything, Mata Ji."

She smiled with that warmth of hers. "Actually it isn't all my idea . . . my son Chandra—the corporal—he thought of a little plan, you see." I nodded again.

"I . . . we all . . . we have seen the beautiful rugs you weave, in the style of your homeland, Tibet. So thick, and soft! And such exotic patterns! And we . . . we know the man in the market who buys them from the Sergeant, you see.

"And my son and I, we went and talked with him; he is really quite well-to-do, you see. And we asked him if he would loan us the money we need to build the addition onto the jail for the children to stay in, and he—he has agreed. And later, you see, he will require . . . eighty of your rugs, to pay back the loan." She looked into my eyes hopefully.

I smiled, and then suddenly it struck me how long it would take me to weave that many extra rugs, on top of the ones I had to do anyway. A lump came into my throat. I didn't know what to say.

"Oh not all by yourself," Mata Ji giggled then, and then took me by the hand. "Come. There are some women here I want you to meet."

And she led me out to the porch, and I saw two ladies seated there, talking softly. One had her back to me, and beyond her the other suddenly looked up, right into my eyes. She was tall, and graceful—older by a bit than Mata Ji, but her face serene and lovely, with noble lines of kindness and thoughtfulness tracing her cheeks and soft brown eyes. She nodded at me with both warmth and nobility, and we stepped towards her.

"This is Amirta, my . . . very close friend. And this, dear Amirta, is of course Miss Friday." And then Mata Ji turned to me with a strange intensity. "You see, Amirta is a widow too, and she too knows the art of weaving, fine weaving. And the two of us, and our other friend, you see, we want to know . . . if you would be kind enough . . . kind enough to teach us how to weave rugs in your beautiful Tibetan style. And then you see, all of us—all of us together—we can make the eighty rugs, and the children, you see . . . they will have a home."

The lady Amirta nodded again, with that high grace, and of course all I could do was nod back—although really I felt like bowing. And then the other woman there, she turned around, and smiled up at me, and said, "And we do hope too that you will let us come and join Mata Ji's classes—the classes on yoga." And I laughed with surprise and nodded again, and held out my hand to the Sergeant's wife.

ɸ

"Fifth and final form of self-control," I announced to the Captain.

"Whew!" he said, with relief.

"Don't be so glad," I warned him. "Three of the others were things we do in our actions: with our bodies. Not such a difficult thing to monitor. The other one, along with . . . " I paused for him.

"Along with its own three friends, are done with our speech: in our words. And the mouth moves pretty fast. Not at all as easy to watch," he said.

"Right," I agreed, painfully aware of that fact. "But now the final form of self-control—which is really three, you see—now *that's* difficult. Because it involves just watching what you *think*—even if the thought never leads you to do or say anything else. And that's a challenge, because a *thought* is the closest thing of all to being a *seed* already."

The Captain squinted, and then got that determined officer's look. "I see what you mean. But if the Master put it among the five, I suppose it's pretty important."

"Just so," I replied. "He says,

> *The fifth form of self-control*
> *Is to overcome possessiveness.*
>
> II.30E

And so at the bottom here is our habit of being possessive— our impulse to acquire, to possess; to control and to own: things, money, people, knowledge, events themselves. We are incapable of finding happiness in any one thing, and so we grasp for more things, imagining that there must be happiness in numbers, or variety, if it cannot be in a single thing.

"This thirst to control, to own, pushes us into two states of mind that we carry around with us all day long. They make us unhappy today, and they plant very powerful seeds to make us unhappy tomorrow. And they are both so very wrong—so very much against the ultimate destiny each one of us has, of becoming a being of light who can help countless people on countless planets. These two states of mind are *so* wrong that they tie up and choke the channels, shoving us daily towards our graves.

"Now the first of these two is that simple, evil emotion of being unhappy whenever someone else gets something nice. I mean, what could be wrong with any single person in this world of death and disappointment coming across even one small happiness, however short-lived it may be? But when we see it happen, our possessiveness rears its ugly head: If happiness is had, it must be mine. And then we feel envy, jealousy—a drive to compete and direct this happiness towards ourselves, like some huge terrible slug that seeks to devour everything in its path.

"Side-by-side with this dismal thought is a second: the satisfaction we feel whenever someone else has a problem, whenever someone else fails. There is the part of us, the part of us all, which stands and stares in fascination as the powerful fall into death or ruin; as the famous struggle and fail to stay on top; as the righteous are tempted and fall. We rush to tell our neighbors, we feel somehow that justice has been done; for it is only ourselves who are exempt from catastrophe, only ourselves who truly never deserve it.

"And so there it is: so hard to face, and so destructive of our own happiness. On any given day, any normal person, all of us, spend much of the time in our own thoughts being unhappy that others are happy, and being happy when others are unhappy—because they possess what we do not, or have lost what only we should possess.

"And behind both these thoughts is the worst one of all: simply misunderstanding our world—really just the pen and the cow. Because, you see, we *cannot* be unhappy with others' happiness, and we *cannot* be happy with their sorrow, if we have even the vaguest comprehension of HOW OUR WORLD REALLY WORKS. There is *no* better way to secure our own misery, now and for years to come, than to be selfish, than to want good things only for ourselves."

"Worldview," said the Captain quietly. "Simply comprehending that every good thing that ever comes to us is literally created by taking care of others. And it is simply beyond the limits of imagination to think of what our world could be like—*will* be like—when people simply figure out that this is the way it all really works."

43

Easy Points

At our next class I wrinkled my forehead, and then tried to smooth it out, but I could tell that the Captain had caught me already. We both smiled.

"One last thing you should know about mental-seed gardening," I said, "and then it's time to go on.

"There are certain kinds of thoughts that are particularly easy for working with seeds; and I mean for either gathering a lot of good ones easily, or destroying a bunch of good ones too, just as quickly. And here we're talking about seeds that also have a particularly fast and powerful effect on your channels.

"If a person for example had a physical problem and was looking to get some help with it by doing yoga, then they'd want to know about the first of these. To do it you simply find a comfortable chair, and sit down for a minute or two, and think about all the good things that someone else is doing.

"It doesn't matter who, really. It could be someone at work; or your husband or wife or someone else in your

337

family; or perhaps some particularly kind person you've only heard about.

"And I'm not saying that you have to pretend that you never see this person get upset sometimes or do perhaps something selfish—that's not the point. We all see that in others, all the time, and it's actually more a statement upon the state of our own seeds.

"But here you just sit down—no need to tell anybody, no need to look like you're doing it—and simply review, carefully, in your mind, all the nice things that someone else is doing, and everything nice about them.

"And I tell you something, Captain—and I have seen this repeated over and over in the ancient books. Whenever we simply sit down and take a few minutes to be *happy* about the good things that someone else is doing—to be happy about the seeds they are planting in their own minds—then *one tenth* of the power of the seeds they have planted, often with a lot of effort over a long period of time, is planted in our *own* minds too."

The Captain arched his eyebrows. "Really? Wonderful! Sort of like the opposite of being glad that someone has a problem. *My goodness*," he said with a smile. "That means that you could just choose some particularly inspiring person—past or present; sit down and be happy about them; and probably plant more good seeds sitting there on your bottom than we usually do for days at a time!"

"I thought you'd like that," I said, and paused for a moment. "But you must also beware of the opposite. There is a kind of thought that can pass through the garden of all the good seeds you have planted in your mind for months and months, and destroy it all in a few minutes, like a hailstorm passing over a field of tender blossoms. And that thought is, quite simply, anger."

The Captain looked up at me quickly, and both of us at the same moment I think saw him standing over me in the cell, with his stick raised. And then it passed, and he gave me that nod that said he had made a note of it, and would not forget.

"To stand and remain without anger in the face of that person or thing which most upsets you has been considered, by the great masters throughout all time, as one of the greatest personal achievements of an entire lifetime. The *Short Book* is speaking of this too when it says,

> *The third commitment*
> *Is facing hardship for higher goals.*
> II.32c"

φ

As always when something is being built there was a steady stream of sweet, big, rough-looking men cursing and spitting and tramping dirt through the jail, asking the corporal where this wall or that wall was supposed to go. Sometimes Long-Life and I would escape out to the front porch for a break, and to play with Busuku's boys.

One day I decided it was time to expand the boys' education beyond just knowing how everything in the world worked; I mean, it's also useful on occasion to be able to write, and all that. And so I came out on the porch and found Young Warrior and took him aside.

"How would you like to learn . . . some other stuff?" I asked.

"What kind of stuff?"

"I mean, things that you would be learning in the town school say; you know, math or science or stuff like that."

Young Warrior gave me sort of a strange look, and then called another boy over. "Rasan," he said. "Did you guys do Red Team, Blue Team yet today?"

The other boy shook his head. "We've been waiting until evening, until all the workers have left."

"Think we could do a little now?"

The other boy glanced at me and said, "You know we're not supposed to show people that game."

"But this is *Miss Friday* we're talking about!" exclaimed Young Warrior.

Rasan looked around, and then broke into a grin. "I suppose we could do just one round, over in the corner of the porch there." And like magic the boys broke off into two lines, sitting facing each other across the porch. Young Warrior got up in the middle, approached one line, and called out "Mathematics."

A thin boy with a big mop of unruly hair threw up his hand.

"How many poles you going for?" demanded Young Warrior.

"The max, of course," declared the boy with bravado.

"It's your neck," answered Warrior, and he paused for a moment to think.

"How much is COUNTLESS?" he blurted then.

"Trick question!" complained the boy. "That's the name of an actual number in the ancient books! Right around ten to the sixtieth power!" he called out confidently, and Young Warrior nodded with a disgruntled look.

And then the boy jumped up and ran around the porch slapping the poles on the four corners, with the other boys yelling and chasing him around some way I couldn't make sense of; and then finally everyone sat back down, and from what I gathered Red Team had scored one "run," and gained one point against the other team.

Young Warrior stood now to face the opposite line of boys. "Physics!" he called, and another thin, tallish boy with raven-black hair falling down across his eyes raised his hand.

"Three poles," he said a little nervously.

"Right," said Warrior, and thought for a moment. "Name any three of the fanciful names given by the ancient Indian physicists to minute particles on the molecular level."

"Oh right, said the boy. "Uh . . . rabbit particles, sheep particles, and . . . uh . . . donkey particles?"

"*Wonk-wonk!*" came a yell from the boys on the other side. The atomic-particle boy jumped up and tried to run to slap the first corner pole, but the other side was up and after him in a flash, and gleefully pulled him back to his seat. No points scored, it seemed. I couldn't believe it.

"Young Warrior; is that stuff for real?"

"Of course," he said blithely. "Master Vasu Bandhu, fourth century, third chapter of his *Treasure House*; and the third one is a *cow* particle, of course, not a donkey!" and he brayed at the boy for good measure.

"Logic!" he called next to the other line of boys. Nobody raised their hand, so Warrior simply pointed at one. "Three forms of valid reasons in a proper syllogism," he said in a tone of mock deadliness. "Worth four poles if you get it," he added brightly.

The boy looked up at the porch roof for help, and some whispers broke out—but were quickly hushed by the other side. Finally the boy sighed loudly and answered, almost helplessly, "Those that involve a result; or identity; or the absence of a thing."

There was a moment of stunned silence and then the boys on his side cheered as one, picked him up on their shoulders, and danced him around to slap the four poles. Somewhere between the second and third pole he hit his head on a roof beam, and gave a tremendous yell, and the other boys dropped him, and the Captain poked his head out the door to call for order, and suddenly they were just a bunch of boys lounging around on a porch again, practicing some yoga poses, chewing some sugar cane.

I looked around in amazement, and said to Young Warrior, "Where . . . how . . . how did you learn those books? And where are the books?"

"Oh, no books," he said with a shy smile. "We had to learn it all in our heads, because we didn't have any money, you see, for books; and we don't know how to write yet either, see, because, well . . . out under the tree . . . in the rain . . . paper and ink, they don't last too long."

"Oh yes, I see," I said quickly. "I'm sure we can work on that now, you see, but . . . but tell me, Young Warrior. *Who taught you all that?*"

"Oh!" he said simply. "It was just Mr. Busuku."

44

The Seer Dwells

Second Week of January

"Mr. Busuku," I called one night to him, softly, more out of habit than for any fear of sticks now.

"Why yes, Miss Friday," came his rascal's voice.

"Mr. Busuku, I . . . well, I heard . . . sort of by accident . . . the boys; they were playing a game, a game of knowledge . . . "

"Ah that," he said quickly. "Nothing, really. Just bits and pieces of stuff I learned a long time ago. Really wish I could have gone on further with them, but feeding them was first priority, and we had trouble getting books and paper, and what-not."

"I see," I said quietly. It didn't feel right to ask him how he had learned the classics—a rare feat for a person of any time in history. And so I simply said, "I think I can get paper, and pens, at least . . . if, if you would like to go on and teach the boys to write."

Busuku was silent for a few minutes and then said, "Miss Friday, I'd be honored to teach the boys to write. But I think too that we should all share the work."

343

"How so?" I said.

He cleared his throat and said, "You see, Miss Friday, I've been giving it a lot of thought, and I don't really approve of the ladies doing all the hard work, and the men getting all the fat jobs. And so I'll agree to teach half the boys writing, but only if *you* agree to put me over in that third cell with the ladies for a few hours a day, and teach me to weave my fair share of the rugs, to help pay for the boys' upkeep. Is that a deal?"

I smiled in the dark. The more I learned about this special little man, the more I realized I'd yet to learn. "A deal, Mr. Busuku, of course, a deal." And then I thought for a moment. "But who's going to teach the *other* half of the boys to write?"

"Ah that," he said, and I could feel his sly grin through the wall. "I suggest you ask Mata Ji's friend—the lady Amirta, you see—but don't let on that I had anything to do with it. Promise?"

"Promise," I replied, more mystified than ever.

φ

Today was a special day, and I sat the Captain down and asked him to pay special attention. "We've pretty much covered all the gardening now," I began. "We went through the five types of self-control, to find out the most powerful ways of making good seeds, and avoiding bad ones. Then we spoke about making good seeds that will never wear out—*higher* good seeds—by thinking about the pen and the cow as you do good things for others; and then also by dedicating what you do, with joy, to the day you will become a being of light that can help every living creature.

"We talked about the four steps for getting rid of *old* bad seeds, and then we spoke of two easy and very powerful ways of either amassing good seeds, or destroying them almost by accident. And so you know really everything you need to know to make a perfect and beautiful garden of your mind and heart. Remember too that keeping some kind of record or diary throughout the day—noting down both your best and worst actions, words, and thoughts—is a completely necessary practical step if you ever hope to collect enough seeds to see things change.

"And you see, things *will* begin to change around you, and I think it's very important that you have some idea of what to expect: things to look forward to, milestones you will reach and pass as you fly towards your final destiny.

"As you advance in your gardening, those three states of mind that we called the 'combined effort' become more and more important . . . " I paused for him to count them back to me.

"The combined effort," he started slowly, like one of Busuku's boys in the porch game. "First, focus: selecting an object and locking your mind on it. Second, fixation: staying on that object over a stretch of time. And then for the third you mentioned 'perfect meditation,' which you said was really just thinking very hard about what's really going on, when you help someone for example."

"Exactly," I said. "And now you need to know that, when your gardening within your own mind gets fairly good, then you will want to practice these three more and more during your silent sitting time.

"The goal at that point is to turn these three more upon your very self: you want to head your thoughts towards discovering your own real nature. This exercise brings you very quickly down a path with some major milestones in your evolution towards becoming someone who can actually help an infinite number of other people at the same time.

"And so, once your gardening is going along pretty well, your channels are already changing: already becoming more pure and free of the choke-points. And you will automatically be drawn to sitting down silently at times and directing the combined effort on your own self.

"And so first you focus on yourself. Then you fix your mind there strongly, in the silence. And then you do that 'perfect meditation' on yourself. The Master describes it like this:

> *Perfect meditation*
> *Then sees this same object*
> *As its simple self:*
> *Its clear light,*
> *Totally void*
> *Of any nature of its own.*
>
> III.3

Now this might sound a little difficult at first, but it's not at all. You already know everything he's talking about here. 'Perfect meditation,' you know, just means a way of looking at something, except now you're doing it during silent sitting. 'This same object' just means whatever thing you have already chosen to focus and fix your mind upon. Before, it was everything involved with helping someone else. Now here it's . . ." I paused.

"Me," he said, "just me, myself."

"Good," I said, and I knew he was still following me closely. "Now when the Master talks about this thing's 'simple self,' what do you suppose he's talking about?"

"From what he says in the few lines after that," said the Captain, "it sounds like he's talking about—let me see, how to put it—it sounds like he's talking about the pen *before* your mind made it a pen, in a way. I mean, it sounds like he's trying to remind us that, at the most basic or simple level of all—the pen in itself is not really even a pen: it's just a green stick that my mind later dresses up as a pen, when seeds go off in my mind and force it to do so."

"Exactly right," I said. "And masters over the centuries have called this most basic or simple level of the pen the 'clear light.' It's not really a kind of physical light, of course; it's simply, you can say, the blank that you draw when you go looking for a pen that could be a pen by itself, from its own side. Sort of like the strong sensation of absence or missingness you get when you have just finished a big meal at a fine restaurant and you reach into your pocket for your wallet to pay the bill, and suddenly realize you left it in your other pair of pants at home."

"*That* is a perfectly clear way to say it," he said. "And I can see how the Master could go on to describe that as a 'total voidness': it's really just that feeling of finding out that something you really thought was there isn't there at all. I mean, I really do strongly remember the day you showed me this idea with the pen: it was such a revolution in my way of seeing things, just to realize that the pen doesn't even have any nature of pen-ness to it, by itself—or else it would be a pen to the cow as well.

"And then when you went that one extra step and explained how it is *seeds* going off in my mind that *do* make *me* see it as a pen, everything tied together so nicely. Because then it gave me real hope, you see, to reach for something even beyond death; to reach my family, really, and more.

Because if the seeds are where things really come from, and if we can *change* the seeds, then *anything* is possible."

"And so you understand what the Master calls 'clear light'; the missing-wallet feeling, but with everything around us—even ourselves. And you see why it's an important part of stopping all the pain in the world. And to grasp these two ideas alone is to reach two very important milestones.

"But I want you to know—and it is the very reason we are speaking today of these things—you must know that, if you continue to make that combined effort in thinking about all this, then there will come a day when you actually *catch your mind* making the pen, or whatever object it may be. I mean, you could be standing at home boiling water in a pot to make some tea. And you are casually looking at the metal pot, but over the past weeks and months you've been thinking very hard about how the seeds make you see things, especially yourself yourself. You've *also* been working very hard on the essence of gardening: you've been trying very hard to be absolutely kind to others.

"And due to the influence of these two on your mind, you see, you suddenly realize that you are not looking at a pot *out there*. You are looking at an impossibly perfect *image* of a pot stitched together by your mind, as the *seeds* to see a pot go off. And your mind is *inserting* this image over some colors and shapes out there that *suggest* a pot.

"And when this happens to you, the day it really happens, you will know that you have reached a milestone. And I remind you that it does not make the pot any less a pot—you will go ahead and finish making your tea in that very same pot: the pot is real; it really works; the tea will taste especially fine that day. It is important then to keep your mind on the main point: how what you have just seen is *proof* that it is possible for every living creature in the world to reach a place beyond all pain, beyond all death.

"And then within that same day you will come to perhaps the greatest milestone of all. It is called the Path of Seeing, and it is so important that the Master describes it in some of the very first lines of his entire book:

> *On that day*
> *The seer comes to dwell*
> *Within their own real nature.*
>
> I.3

What we call Seeing here, it always happens during your silent sitting, just after that milestone with the pot that we talked about. And you go deep within your mind, and you see something very deep about yourself. All your other thoughts stop: you can't see or hear anything outside, and even inside you are no longer even thinking 'I'm seeing something special now.' You just *see*.

"And what you *see* is your own real nature. Oh not with your eyes, of course, and not even with your regular kinds of thoughts. Because *those* kinds of thoughts, you see, are always mixed up with misunderstanding things: with feeling that what they are comes from them. And so for almost all of us—even those who understand what it is to *misunderstand*—the misunderstanding goes on all the time, at a very deep level, whenever we are simply perceiving the things around us, or even just thinking.

"In terms of those channels deep within us—in terms of the subtle winds within them then—the two side channels are always full and bulging with thoughts of misunderstanding, and the two poisons that are born from it: liking things in a mistaken way, and disliking things in a mistaken way. And then flowing with these thoughts flies a swarm of others. In the channel of the moon, thoughts of possessiveness, impossible desires, pride: all related to that stupid kind of liking. In the channel of the sun, thoughts of anger, hatred, competition: all related to that stupid kind of disliking.

"But on the day that you *see*, you see—in that brief period of *seeing*, which lasts for less than half an hour; at that most blessed milestone of all—then for those few precious minutes *all* the misunderstanding is stopped. *All* the power of the winds in the side channels is *stopped*. And then the seer, you see—the person who is *seeing*, seeing the clear light raw, as it is—he or she can stop and *dwell* there, in what is their own real nature. They are not just *understanding* that the pen is not a pen from its own side: they are *dwelling* in the ultimate nature of the pen.

"And you see, all the things around us, including even ourselves—all of them put together are something that we call our reality: our world, everything we know. But on the day that you *see*, you reach a completely different reality—an infinitely higher reality. And it is clear and pure and invisible and ultimate as only a diamond is within our usual reality: completely clear and colorless; purely diamond within every atom of the diamond; and in its own poor physical way a metaphor for what is ultimate, since no object within this universe can scratch a diamond, but for another diamond. And you *dwell* in this higher reality, for those few minutes, and the only wind and thought within you with any strength at that time is the *seeing*, and it lies only in the middle channel, for the first time of all.

"And then you stir yourself from the seeing, and with this the winds in the side channels are stirred once again, and you leave the place where you have dwelled. But it is a milestone, you see—for if the winds move like that, purely and totally, only within the middle channel, if even for only those few minutes, then you are changed forever; and you are very close to becoming that being of perfect light who can go to help countless others on countless planets, all at once, as is each of our destiny.

"And in the hours after *seeing*, in that same day itself, you see into the future, and you see, and you *know*, the being that you will become; and you *know* when it will be, with total surety. And on this day too the knot at the heart will be opened, and you will experience, for the first time, the full form of that joy we talked about: you *see* the infinite number of living creatures upon every world of the universe *directly*; and you know that you will work to help and serve them, forever; and you first see, directly, those who have gone before you to this same high goal. And so that is the seeing, of the Master's seer, and I so much wanted you to hear of it, and know that it is coming to you, and to all who tend that most sacred garden, of their own mind."

45

Time and Space, Reduced to a Puddle

Third Week of January

The day of the celebration—I will never forget it; it was a Friday. We worked hard to finish up all our regular tasks before noon. Mata Ji and the Sergeant's wife, working in the third cell, tied off four new rugs for market. Amirta and Busuku had to give double classes to the boys, since the Sergeant—who had taken upon himself all the duties of a school principal—absolutely refused to consider their missing the afternoon lesson. The corporal spent the entire morning out in front balanced precariously on a tall ladder that he drafted the Captain to hold for him. When they were finished they ran inside like two little schoolboys, and made us all come out to see.

The royal insignia—the image of a lion and crossed swords scratched into the mud on the front of the station—had been replaced by a huge new wooden sign. It was still a lion—but he was standing on his two hind legs now, and holding up a cushion. On top of the cushion was a child, seated in the Lotus Pose, with a book open upon his lap. And the swords were gone.

"The new wave!" declared the corporal proudly.

"Doing things with understanding, and not with sticks or steel!" crowed the Captain. And we all stood for a good long time and ooh-ed and ah-ed and enjoyed the glow of the change that the sign itself marked in our lives.

And then by afternoon all the boys were scrubbed and dressed in their new white cottons, and the corporal had finished mopping the entire station for the third time, and even the Captain's lair was neat as a pin. Mata Ji and her crew arrived with piles of freshly cooked dishes, and Busuku produced a massive fruit salad he'd made himself ("Not fair to let the ladies have all the fun cooking").

The construction men and their families had been invited to help open the new wing, and they brought flutes and pretty little drums with them. Even the shop owner who had loaned the money showed up; he brought a huge platter of sweets, and after seeing what a wonderful thing was happening he let the corporal talk him into cutting the interest on the loan down by six rugs.

And so we opened all the cells to make room for everyone and we ate and laughed and planned a glorious future, and at some point the builders got up and started to dance. It was a simple country dance in pairs with their womenfolk, and it made me homesick for the bonfire dances of my little village back in Tibet. At some point Busuku got up and said loudly, "I think Miss Friday should have a chance to see our country's classical dance!"

Everyone murmured in agreement; Busuku raised his hands in high drama. "And although I myself am a veritable expert at the ancient dance, I am . . . still rather sore from Miss Friday's torture . . . ah, I mean *yoga class* of this morning. Fortunately though, I am aware that there is one among us who once studied this priceless tradition.

And I call upon him, or her, to stand and dance, in honor of our people's timeless glory."

Another excited murmur passed through the party; everyone looked at everyone else, but no one moved. Busuku stood where he was, his belly—well now sort of a *barrel* really—thrust forward and his hands solid on his hips. "Come now! Don't be shy! Goodness, everyone has been studying Master Patanjali's *Short Book* so faithfully, and no one pays him any respect! *Red Team!*" he roared.

"Yes *sir!*" yelled back a gaggle of his boys.

"History!"

"Sir!" they yelled again.

"Master Patanjali is recognized as the forefather of four great arts. Name them!"

"Philosophy—especially the philosophy of yoga!" called out one boy.

"Medicine!" added another, quickly.

"The science of the Mother Tongue," came a third.

"And last, but not least... " Young Warrior got up and waved his arms and wiggled his hips, "our country's classical dance!"

The crowd burst out into laughter, and next to me the Captain leaned over and whispered, "Is that... is that true?"

"What's that?" I said.

"The Master—is he really considered a forefather of each of these arts?"

"Why yes," I replied, "as well he should! Those who master yoga master yoga because they care for others, and that explains the medicine. And the Mother Tongue, from which so many languages of the world have sprung, sings within our very channels as yoga helps us open them. And as they open we feel so light and full of cheer that—well— we are nearly *compelled* to dance!"

The Captain turned to me, his eyes aglow. "A fire I feel inside of me, at this very moment."

And he rose, and faced Busuku across the circle, and said, "Sir! I know not how you could have learned that I once studied at the feet of the master dancers of our great capital, however briefly . . . ," and he looked down quickly for a moment.

And then his eyes came up again, glistening now, and he sang, "And so, in honor of the Master; for all that we have been so blessed to learn . . . ," and he took off his beautiful red sash and the pure white shirt, and set them at my side, and removed his shoes, and stepped to the middle of the circle.

And the flutes began, and then later the drums joined in, and at first he was a cobra, moving slow and sinuous from side to side. And then the music changed and he was like a deer, flying first here, and then there, in graceful bounds and leaps. And then finally as dusk itself set outside the music changed to something dark, and powerful, and he was up on his toes with his arms and head thrown to the sky, like an eagle drinking lightning from the clouds. And there was a great crescendo and the sweat was cascading down his chest and over us from his fingers and he was whirling and . . .

The music suddenly stopped. A huge, dark figure filled the doorway, his impossibly broad shoulders touching the frame on each side. He took one step inside—the last red rays of sunlight pouring in from the windows in the back caught his face: a face of power and strength, a strong straight nose of nobility, steel eyes and short-cut curls of steel silver hair.

The Captain turned, his chest heaving for breath, and caught the man's eyes full. "Sir!" he said only.

"Captain!" the man replied. "Captain Kishan!" And there was a tiny moment of silence in the near dark of the room.

"Into your room, Captain!" ordered the Superintendent then. "You have . . . some explaining to do, I think."

φ

For three days we saw little of the Captain. The Superintendent showed up with several guards, usually in the afternoon, and then alone went straight to the Captain's office and closed the door. Whatever words they shared were so soft that we could never catch them listening at the wall; but so intense that we couldn't ignore them either.

Everyone was on pins and needles. The Sergeant kept the boys off in the addition, with minimum classes. The weavers stayed home and did what they could from there. Busuku was so nervous it seemed that he fell ill and passed all day every day flat on his bed with the covers thrown over his head. The corporal spent most of his time out back with a motley collection of abandoned animals, trying hopelessly to keep them from mooing, oinking, and cackling. On the fourth day, in the morning, the Captain called me in.

"Miss Friday, my Teacher . . . ," he began, looking a little preoccupied. "I thought . . . I thought that perhaps, if you agree, we could . . . we could continue our classes as usual, despite the circumstances. And I want the boys to continue too, out in the front room. Even in the so-called normal times of our lives, we never know when something might strike suddenly to end whatever chance we have to do something important, like our yoga together. And as things stand here now, at the station—I'm afraid life is even less certain than usual. So I would like to continue the classes, for everyone, with every moment we have left to us."

I nodded. "Of course," I said. We were silent for a time, and then I added, "Are things going that badly?"

The Captain looked me straight in the eye, and then looked down again. "To tell you the absolute truth, I can't figure out *how* things are going. The Superintendent is playing his cards very close to his chest. I mean, from the very first night . . . I was very clear to him, I was very honest. I tried *so hard* to be aware of the seeds I was planting, because I feel like the present moment is somehow very important—very crucial—and that something strong can happen if I follow the self-control right now very purely, very closely.

"And so I have been totally honest with the Superintendent, about what I did in the past, and about what we are all doing here now. And he listens very carefully, and he asks me many questions about then and now; and he seems somehow to know a lot about life at our station of late. But like anyone skilled in the politics of the royal court, he keeps his feelings from his face—for now. It feels as though he is deciding something, and I honestly cannot tell what that may be."

I nodded in sympathy, and we were quiet for another moment. "But one more thing," he added then, with no little sadness in his voice.

"What's that?" I asked.

He drew himself up taller, and spoke slowly, his voice tight with emotion. "It is your case," he said then softly. "The Superintendent has agreed to hear your case. In fact, he will hear it later today, in the afternoon." The Captain turned his eyes up to me, and they were moist, and suddenly I felt my own fill with tears. The school—the jail—I realized then that it had become my home. I realized that it had not been a jail at all to me for the past many months.

But there was nothing to say of it—we had to see what our seeds would bring to us. And so I simply replied "I see," in a voice that told him where my home was, and then cleared my throat and began the class, as all classes should begin: as if it very well might be the last.

"We have been talking of milestones," I reminded him, "that will surely come to you as you continue the gardening of your mental seeds. And today I thought we should speak about milestones in how you see your own mind change.

"Because, you see, the way you see *your own mind* is no more something that comes from its own side than the pen. What I mean to say is that—as with the pen—your mind picks up certain indications, as you listen to your own thoughts. And then seeds from how you treated others in the past go off, you see, and determine even what *your own thoughts* will sound like to *yourself:* just like the pen.

"And you see, if you keep up the various forms of self-control, steadily and sincerely, over a good period of time, then the seeds in your own mind make you *hear* your own thoughts in a completely different way. They begin to sound sweeter and sweeter; more and more pure, with each passing day—and it's a true pleasure then to simply *be* within your own mind.

"And there will come a day—that glorious day— when you hear your own mind think its last tiny echo of a negative thought, and then those thoughts will simply fade forever into silence. Try to imagine it: not a few minutes, or an hour, or even a whole day spent without anger or jealousy or pride—but rather *the rest of time itself* in a pure contentment forever free of those thoughts. The last to go is the misunderstanding itself; and there comes a day when nothing in your entire world ever again appears as if it were itself by itself, from its own side."

"Sounds simple, but for *nothing* at all around us, in our entire life, to even *suggest* being something from its own side—I imagine that must be something extraordinary," said the Captain.

"Oh yes," I said, "I imagine so." And it left us in silence for a while. "But then the mind goes further," I went on. "Radical changes begin to occur in the channels, and the winds, and the thoughts that ride them, and the mind itself. And it is all in preparation—it is all building up to the day that your body itself transforms into living crystal, living light, and you gain the power you were meant to have—to appear on all worlds, before all living creatures, in whatever way most fits their needs of every moment.

"And you see, just before this last thing happens—in the single split-second before this happens—your mind suddenly reaches the power to know all the things there are, and all that ever were, or will be, anywhere: and you know all these things in an instant, and for all time to come.

"And today I felt—I mean, even if we were never to speak together again at all—I felt that you should hear this thing from me. And it is the tradition of our lineage—it is the way of all the Masters who have passed this knowledge down, from Teacher to pupil, from century to countless century—that you must not only *hear* that your mind will gain this power; you must *understand* why your mind will gain this power, for in understanding it the power is surely come.

"And really, it goes back simply to the pen. The Master says it this way:

> *It comes because*
> *Those who understand things*
> *Have broken through the idea*
> *That past and future*
> *Are times that could exist*
> *In and of themselves.*

IV.12

It's really not a difficult idea at all," I said. "The pen's being a pen . . . " I paused.

"Doesn't come from its own side. It comes from mine, from my own mind, as seeds ripen there to make me see it that way."

"And *time*, you see—*time* itself is THE SAME." I locked my eyes to his, almost to give it to him through our eyes. "The past is not *past* from its own side. The future is not *future* from its own side. We look at time itself: we look at events as they happen to us, and then our mind—*and it is only our mind*—splits this up into the ever-moving present moment, and the past, and the future to come.

"And you see—again—it is only the seeds going off within our own minds that make us see time this way, split into three. If we had *different* seeds, then time—*all the time there ever was, or will be* — would be for us only a single *point*, and not a flow divided into three parts. And then we could—we will—simply gaze upon that single point, and see all. Stand in the middle of a huge city, like the capital—and in a single moment see the city thriving; the city being built; the last brick of the city falling to the ground; countless cities that stood on that ground before; countless cities that will stand on that ground again; the ground itself forming from the dust of stars; the ground itself melting into air at the touch of a star; and countless stars themselves—come, gone, shining, dark: all in a single instant.

"Every mind that is alive at this moment on every planet there is, regardless of the body it dwells within now—human, animal, bird, insect—all minds will one day have the power to see this, to see time as a single point. For it is what our minds are really meant to be: it is what all minds grow into, after the infancy we live in now is finished.

"And that's not all, you see. Because whatever is true of the true nature of time is equally true of the true nature of space itself: of *place*, of *distance*. Which is to say the fact that the wall is *far* from us, and your desk is *close* to us—this fact too cannot be coming from its own side, any more than the pen can. It too is an image created by seeds ripening within the mind, and would be—will be—different if the seeds are different. All that is far could be where all that is near is now: all place there is could be—will be—a single place, a single point, when your seeds are perfect; when you finish the gardening. And then, you see, there is nothing in the universe, wherever it may be, that you do not see, in a single moment, in a single place. The Master says it like this:

> *When knowledge is no longer blocked,*
> *Then all there is to know*
> *Is reduced to the size of a puddle.*
> IV.31B"

We sat then in silence again, knowing that events were in motion that could keep the two of us in silence, and content somehow nonetheless. Then finally the Captain stirred and said, "But—if I may ask—what kind of action could it be that we do towards others, which could ever plant such seeds in the first place: seeds to see time broken up, with almost all of it out of our reach; seeds to see place itself broken the same way, and nearly all of it far from us?"

"It is quite simple," I began slowly, "and quite sad. These things have been removed from us because we have removed ourselves from others. These seeds were planted, and continue to be planted, simply by seeing others as something *different* from ourselves.

"And oh, I don't mean that somehow we are everybody else and they are us. That is not the way it is, and it will never be that way, simply because of the way that seeds—even the highest seeds—themselves work. You see—and I think it must have occurred to you by now—I cannot plant a seed for you, and you cannot plant one for me. No matter how far along we may go, and no matter how much we may love others, we cannot add or subtract an iota from their seeds.

"And that is why we cannot simply take away another person's pain, and it also explains why we ourselves still *have* pain. Because surely, if it were at all possible, then the great ones who have gone before us would have taken away our pain already. And so I cannot *become* you in that sense, for you are and always will be only the result of what you yourself have planted, as you were kind or not to others.

"But we *can*, and we *must*, remove the idea of any difference between ourselves and others on a completely different level. I mean, the great error of humankind which has kept us constantly in misery, since our kind began—and which has planted the seeds that restrict us to time itself, and to a single place—is that we separate our happiness from the happiness of others. We *decide* to work for one—we make the decision to spend our entire lives, and every single effort of those lives, working for one—and we *decide* that the other is not as important, or perhaps not important at all.

"And so you see, this one decision—this one simply arbitrary decision to split ourselves from others, by splitting our happiness away from their happiness—it causes the very division of time as we know it, into past and present and future. And it creates the reality of distance between the things around us. And by doing so it locks us into a tiny terrible jail of a body like this, locked into a small dangerous world, locked into a flow of time that will sweep us away to the ugly terrors of old age and then to death itself.

"And if we would be free of all this—as we all wish to be, deep inside—then we need only take the first step, to do small things for others: to try to remove the division into *their* happiness or *my* happiness. And that all begins with never hurting others to get what we want. It begins with those precious forms of self-control, and expands to doing the opposite—to helping others, to serving others—until the day we become what we have really always been striving to become: a being whose eyes are no longer limited by time, nor even by space, in the service of others."

φ

In the afternoon the Sergeant came solemnly to my door and made a show of removing the crossbar, with the Superintendent's guards looking on from the front of the jail. His boy Ajit was already there, and I too made a point of telling him in front of the guards that the Captain wanted classes to resume as normal, starting today. And then I walked to the Captain's room, escorted closely by both the Sergeant and the corporal. We were all so nervous. Things had changed so quickly.

The Superintendent was seated behind the Captain's desk, but on a much higher cushion. The Captain himself sat nervously to the far side. The Sergeant and the corporal softly shut the door, sat me down before the desk, and took their places off to my left. The Superintendent's massive chest and shoulders were themselves intimidating, even before he spoke a word, and he set his eyes upon me gravely.

"Ah yes, now, then may I declare this court in order," he said in a deep bass voice, deadly serious. "Captain Kishan present to deliver any necessary additional testimony; his two officers in attendance as witnesses. And the accused, a—" he looked down at some notes before him, "a Miss Friday, a foreigner, charged with attempting to enter the borders of the Realm with valuable contraband; and further charged with attempted escape from a government correctional facility." He cleared his throat again, and narrowed his eyes at me.

"May I tell you first, Miss Friday, that the charges against you are quite serious. And despite certain information I have received personally from the Captain regarding this case, I must still inform you that—should you be found in any way guilty of either of these charges today—you face an extended sentence in one of the long-term prisons in the capital. And this facility is a heaven compared to them, I assure you. I therefore encourage you to simply admit your guilt and submit yourself to the leniency of this court, and I tell you truthfully that I will do my best to mitigate your punishment."

I sat up straight and raised my head the way Grandmother would have. "I understand your offer, and I thank you gratefully. But insofar as I bear no guilt at all in these matters, but rather have been held here for nearly a full year without proper recourse to an official such as yourself, invested with the power of examining my case and duly releasing me, then I simply request that you proceed, in due accordance with the law of the Realm." He raised his eyebrows. "Thank you," I added, as Grandmother would have done.

"How old *are* you?" he asked.

"Eighteen, sir," I replied. He raised his eyebrows again, and then pulled out that precious cloth with the Master's ever-so-precious *Short Book*.

"And you, at your age, and a mere girl—you claim that this ancient book is your own, and that you are fully conversant with the Mother Tongue, in which it is written?"

"It *is* my book," I replied with power, "and yes, though but a mere . . . *girl*," my eyes flashed, "I read it as well . . . or *better* . . . than any *man*." And my look dared him to prove otherwise.

His own eyes sparked briefly, and he opened the book's cover with his two huge hands. And then, as the Captain had done on that first day, he flipped the book open to a page at random and stabbed his finger at a line.

"There," he demanded. "Those words—what they say, and what they mean."

I looked and closed my eyes and saw Katrin reading the line to me:

> *"The fourth commitment*
> *Is to regular study.*
>
> II.32E

And what it *means* is that any person who hopes to gain the real results of yoga must commit themselves to serious and constant study of how it works. And this means formal study, with a teacher who really knows the deeper ideas behind things like the yoga poses and breathing exercises. It means establishing a true connection to the countless Masters of the past, by meeting them directly in their own great books; spending time to think out their ideas, and how they apply to our own lives; and gaining from a living teacher the insights upon these ideas passed down as the experience of real people, from generation to generation."

The Superintendent's eyes widened ever so slightly—
but then he simply moved his finger back slightly and said,
"Now these words."

I glanced and closed my eyes and heard Katrin, again.

"The second commitment
Is to be contented
With whatever we have.

II.32B

It is a commitment to be content with what we have—although *never* with what we could become. Because, you see,
no one has all the circumstances they need to practice yoga
and all its ideas. Things are never perfect. It is always too hot,
or too cold. The body is always hurting somewhere; the mind
is always tired or sad. And there is always someone nearby
who disturbs us. Time itself is always short, and we must
always make do with what we have. None of the great ones
who followed this path before us — *none* of them, over the
centuries—possessed perfect circumstances either. And so
they just worked hard with what they had available to them,
and they reached their ultimate goals. Thus one who fol-
lows this way commits to be contented — contented with the
food, contented with the place, contented with the weather,
contented with the current condition of body and mind, contented with the company. And they do not sacrifice a single
moment of their short, precious lives to the poison of com-
plaining—out loud or in their thoughts—about anything."

The Superintendent glanced uncomfortably over to
the Captain and then, less surely now, opened the book to
another page, setting his finger upon a line.

"Theirs is won through effort.

I.20B

366

Here the Master is talking about people who seek goals that are higher than just pleasure or happiness of the kind that cannot last. And he says that they win their goals through *effort:* but it is not effort in the common sense of the word. For it appears here in a list of mighty deeds known as the Five Powers, and as such it refers to *what we enjoy:* what we delight in working towards, even if the work is hard. And so most people would endure any hardship, over their entire lifetime, to earn *money.* And with it they acquire what they *enjoy:* a nice house, pleasant meals, an occasional night out for some entertainment; things like that. But those who grasp how deadly simple life will always be; those who really see the pain around them and ahead of us all; their idea of what is enjoyable changes completely. They would rather spend a night alone in contemplation of how to remove the pain of people, than attend a party to talk to people all dying unknowing. Their idea of entertainment is to go to a hospital to visit the sick. The food they enjoy is only whatever would make them light and strong and healthy to serve others, and not what is sweetest or most expensive. In short, enjoyment is for them the joyful hard work it takes to take care of others."

The Superintendent laid his hand thoughtfully down on the book, and considered for a moment. Then he raised his eyes and leveled them again upon my own. "I tell you truthfully, my young woman, that you speak with a grace far beyond your years. And this is something which the Captain also said of you." And then he was silent again.

"But you see," he said finally, "it is all so . . . I mean . . . it is all, to be honest, only . . . *circumstantial,* you see. You speak well; but frankly, thieves have been known to speak well too. And you must know that *we* cannot read the book. We have no idea if anything you have said so well is really there at all." And then he paused again.

"The Captain says . . . that you claim to have received the book from . . . from a teacher?" he asked.

"From my teacher Katrin," I said, and the memory of it brought tears to my eyes, to match my growing sense of frustration, and even fear.

"And this . . . Katrin . . . is the one who taught you these things?" he asked again, a little more gently.

"Yes," I said, lowering my head, ashamed for them to see me weep. "Katrin, and my uncle, Uncle Jampa."

"And how did *they* learn them?"

"Here," I said in a small voice. "Here in India; they studied . . . they studied where I was headed before . . . before I was arrested, you see: they studied in the holy city of Varanasi, on the banks of the Mother Ganges."

"Hmm," mused the Superintendent. "And so you . . . you retrace their steps, which no doubt took them through the Realm itself." And then he looked intently in my face and added, quickly, "Your uncle—what did you say his name was again?"

"It is Jampa, sir; he is my Uncle Jampa." I was almost whimpering, and it made me more ashamed still.

"Oh yes, Jampa . . . but I mean, in our language—or in the Mother Tongue—in *our* language, what would his name be?" he hurried on.

"Oh, I don't know, let me see, sir . . . in the Mother Tongue, well . . . his name, Jampa, you see—it would be . . . it would be *Maitri.*"

The Superintendent's jaw dropped. "*Maitri!*" he exclaimed. "*Maitri Pandita!*" And then suddenly from the other side of the wall came another loud "*Maitri Pandita!*"

The Superintendent's head jerked up, and he stared at the Captain. "What's that?" he asked.

The Captain looked embarrassed. "Oh nothing sir, nothing at all. My apologies. A prisoner, you see . . . a strange man, you see, yells a lot . . . "

"Odd," said the Superintendent, with his head still up and his ear cocked; and then he recollected himself and brought his eyes back to my own.

"Goodness, girl. Are you . . . are you claiming to be the niece of the *Maitri Pandita*, the greatest wise man this Realm has ever seen?"

"I don't know," I said. "Though I am . . . I am Uncle Jampa's niece; yes I am," I replied, silly with fear and hope. But the Superintendent was overcome with excitement.

"It was in the days of the old King; a great master of yoga came through, and visited the court. He even taught the King, and there were lessons—private lessons; oh, they were so wonderful, for the Crown Prince, bless his soul, and I was there too, and Captain—your own uncle, you see— this is where he started, this was how he began to learn. And the Maitri Pandita, you see, he was a Tibetan; and he had gained knowledge in Varanasi; and he was on his way back home, and he was looking for someone, someone he had lost, and so he came to the King for help . . . "

The Superintendent glowered at me one last time. "Who would he have been looking for? Answer me true, girl, for the rest of your life depends on it."

I smiled in relief. "That would surely have been my aunt," I replied. "His sister."

"And her name?" came the final demand.

I burst out crying, with love of her memory. "You . . . you would have known her name . . . as *Dakini*."

The Superintendent's face suddenly twisted in emotion, and tears sprang from his eyes. He struggled to his feet; the

Captain rushed forward to help him; the Sergeant and the corporal sprang up; the corporal slipped and fell right back down on his bottom. The Superintendent stepped around the desk and enveloped me in his huge arms.

"Maitri Pandita!" he cried, "Maitri Pandita! The niece of the Maitri Pandita! Oh my! Oh my goodness!" And his chest heaved and his tears poured down on my head, and then we were laughing and crying together, still in each other's arms.

"Guards!" roared the Superintendent, and the door burst open almost instantly.

"Sir!" they cried in unison.

"Run to town! Get some sweet tea ... get some fine pastries ... some delicious fruit! Run! First man back wins a gold coin, by goodness!" They were gone in a blink, without stopping even to close the door.

And then the Superintendent sat down and began to wring my hands in his (it hurt!) and cried some more and begged my forgiveness, and I said it was nothing and he told me he would arrange a villa in town with three or four servants to wait on me, and I said I really preferred the jail, and the Captain sat up proudly at that. And then through the open door we heard Busuku's boys get up from their silent sitting—giving and taking—and Ajit was getting them lined up for their poses, and the Superintendent asked what it was and we said their yoga practice, and he started crying again and blubbered on about the old days and the classes with the Maitri Pandita, who he missed so much, and ...

"Rasan! Suck in that lunch box, for goodness sake!" came a shrill yell from the back.

The Superintendent froze. There was a tense silence. He shook his head and said "Can't be" to himself but he got up quickly, motioned to the Captain to remain where he was, and went swiftly to the door. I looked at the Sergeant and the corporal, and we all just shrugged, and then got up to follow the Superintendent out. He stepped slowly through the boys, to the back of the jail—to the bars of Busuku's cell. The three of us huddled behind him. Busuku was back in bed, with the blanket over his head.

"You there," said the Superintendent. "You."

The edge of the blanket came up the tiniest bit, and I knew Busuku was peeking out at the Superintendent's massive feet.

"You," called the Superintendent.

"*Sick*," groaned Busuku in an odd voice, and pulled the blanket down tighter around his head.

"Take off the blanket," said the Superintendent.

"Sick . . . "

The Superintendent whirled around. "Sergeant!"

"Sir!"

"Instruct the prisoner to remove the blanket, or remove it for him."

"Busuku . . . ," pleaded the Sergeant, but his hands never moved to the crossbar. I glanced over then and saw that he had already sawed it in two for Busuku—probably as a gift, on the day of the party. I tried to crowd in between the Superintendent and the crossbar so he wouldn't notice it, and the Sergeant glanced at me gratefully.

"Busuku," he said again, urgently; and then an idea came to him.

"Corporal," said the Sergeant. "Bring your stick—we'll just poke him and wake him up."

The corporal froze, and gave the Sergeant a look that said he had no idea where his stick was. The Sergeant shot back a panicked look that said he had gotten rid of his again. They both thought of the Captain's dusty stick at the same time, propped up in the corner of his office.

"Be right back, sir!" and they turned and rushed to the Captain's office.

Busuku peeked out, threw off the blanket, and turned to face the Superintendent.

The Superintendent straightened suddenly in shock, and gasped—"Your Highness!" There was an unreal moment of silence, and then the Sergeant and corporal came running back, both wielding the single stick high in the air with both hands.

"Your *Slyness!*" roared Busuku, with a mighty laugh. "That's a good one, Big Man! Nobody's called me that *in years!* People around here, see, they all just call me *Busuku,* you see—Mr. Worthless I am—and I kinda *prefer* the name, do you see?" He looked significantly at the Superintendent.

"As you wish," said the Superintendent then, and he turned slowly, and walked back to the Captain's room, deep in thought—and he hardly seemed to taste the pastries when they arrived.

46

Standing on the River

Fourth Week of January

A few days later the Sergeant came to the door of my cell, open now free, and said to me quietly, "Miss Friday, something odd . . . I hope everything is all right. But the Superintendent, you see—he says he must take testimony . . . about . . . about the condition of the jail here; he has called a few other people too . . . he says he needs testimony from the prisoners, and people who were here, and saw what was going on . . . " He looked quite upset. "I just hope . . . I just hope that the Captain will be all right, you see," and he wiped away a tear from his eye.

"So please come along," he said then quietly, "to the porch . . . Superintendent, he says that . . . the three of us . . . are confined to the Captain's room, while he takes the testimony."

He led me to the front door. The Superintendent was standing just outside; he took me lightly by the arm and nodded to the Sergeant, who retreated to the Captain's office. I saw that the side of the porch had been partitioned off with several large sheets of colored cloth, to make a screen all

373

round. Out front, in the corporal's lovely little garden, the Superintendent's usual guards—and some more soldiers too—were sitting around incongruously among the dainty blossoms. Their swords were unsheathed and close at hand; they made a pretense of talking as they scanned the road outside. Something was going on.

The Superintendent led me to the partition, and we ducked under. Inside sat Busuku and Mata Ji's friend, Amirta. And then suddenly the Superintendent was down on his knees, bowing and touching his forehead to Busuku's feet.

"Crown Prince," he said softly, and I could feel the tears coming in him again. "Prince Dabi, Your Highness. So many years. So long, without knowing if you were dead or alive. Oh, it is a wonder, and a blessing, to be in your royal presence again."

And then Busuku reached out and placed his hand gently upon one huge shoulder, with noble affection, and said quietly, "Jaya, my dear friend; loyal to us then, loyal to us now; loyal to the old King, my dear father, loyal to the new King, my dear younger brother. You have served well; you serve well; may you always serve well."

And then he gently urged the Superintendent to stand, and he did, but just as quickly threw himself down before the lady Amirta. "Queen Mother," he sighed simply, and sobbed there at her feet.

She too touched his shoulder, and said only "Splendid Jaya, splendid man," and motioned him to sit. I stood there stunned, too stunned to move.

"Why sit yourself down, Miss Friday," grinned Busuku . . . or the Crown Prince.

"She . . . she is your *mother?*" I stammered.

Amirta glanced over at Busuku with a mischievous smile. "Miss Friday certainly means that I look far too young; or you too old," she explained, and took my hand gently, and sat me down beside her, and held my hand then warmly.

"Prince Dabi," she said to Busuku, "I believe we have some explaining to do to our two—rather confused—friends."

"Ah yes," he said cheerfully. "But where to begin?" he screwed up his face and thought for a minute. "It is quite some time since your dear Uncle, the beloved Maitri Pandita, passed through our Realm," he said to me. "Nearly thirty years, in fact. And it is more than twenty years since my father, the old King, passed away—and the struggle for the throne broke out.

"We never expected any of it; the Queen Mother and I were caught unawares by one of the factions, and spirited away from the palace in the dark of night. They rode us west for days, until we met up with a chieftain of one of the Kashmiri tribes, and we were turned over to be killed, or sold as slaves."

"Ah, but my son's golden tongue saved us from either ignominy," smiled the Queen Mother.

Busuku blushed . . . sort of. "I suppose so," he allowed. "At any rate, I convinced the man that he could get a lot more money if he allowed me some time to arrange a ransom from influential friends back home."

"And so he held us, and kept us alive, and fairly well treated," continued the Queen Mother.

"And each time the ransom was raised, he simply raised the ransom," laughed Busuku. "Three years he lived off us! And then finally we just escaped . . . "

" . . . and came here, to this town on the border of our Realm," finished the Queen Mother.

"And we learned, of course, that my younger brother had succeeded in winning back the throne, and returned the Realm to a state of relative peace," said Busuku. "And so we paused, Mother and I, because we had an idea—we had a vision: something we had talked of frequently during our capture; something that your uncle, Miss Friday, had inspired within the two of us.

"And the idea was this. Knowing that the throne was in good hands, the Queen Mother and I were free—*really* free, for the first time—to try to make some changes in our country, but from the *bottom*; from the grass roots."

"Our vision," continued the Queen Mother, "was to rule from the *bottom*, while my younger son ruled from the top."

"Yes," said Busuku with obvious excitement. "You see, it is one thing to *impose* rule upon a people, even if it is a just and gentle rule. But it is a completely *different* thing to be among the people themselves—to live among people, to listen to people, to experience their joy and their troubles—and then go about improving their lives, within their lives."

"But we needed something concrete to *give* the people, you see," said the Queen Mother, just as excited. "We wanted more than just food in every belly. We wanted more than just a cow and a horse tied to a little house, for each family. We wanted *more* for our people than just mediocre prosperity and then the usual quiet, violent descent of every one of them into old age, and death. To put it briefly, we loved our people, as the old King had taught us to love them: and he loved them too much not to try to give them real happiness—a happiness beyond things to eat and things to buy—a happiness that would *last*, and make them . . . well . . . really *happy*."

"And so we started, just with little things, on a small scale, you see," went on Busuku. "We had learned some things from your uncle that we thought we would try to implement . . . "

"But soon we realized two facts," said the Queen Mother. "First, that these things take time, years of time: planning; night-and-day devotion; and training—building hearts and building people. Secondly, and it took us years to see it, we realized that we needed to know more about *how* the yoga your uncle had taught us really worked."

"And it was around then . . . ," said Busuku, looking at the Superintendent.

The Superintendent's eyes lit up. "Ah!" he said, and then smiled and shook his head in wonder. "It was around then, that I begin getting odd, inspired, and inspiring letters from an anonymous party, obviously educated at court, and obviously in sympathy with the new King and the idea of building a better kingdom—not from the top or the outside but from within the minds of the people themselves.

"And the plan is laid out so clearly and with such conviction that I decide to go along with it, and thus I have, for all these years; beginning with finding a young man who already has seeds in him for the way of yoga, and who can be sent to this town on some pretext to serve in a government post. Someone to be built into a leader — into a teacher — without even knowing he is being built."

"The Captain!" I exclaimed.

"Ah please, Miss Friday," said Busuku wryly. "The walls have ears, and some parts of our plan must remain, shall we say, a mystery until the proper time."

"But then there was . . . a bit of a delay . . . ," suggested the Queen Mother. Busuku looked a little annoyed.

"Not really a *delay*, Mother. Just sort of a . . . well, shall we say . . . an extended *learning experience*."

"You see," she went on, "the Crown Prince . . . he slowly became aware of all the children in the town who had no parents, and no homes, and no one to take care of them. And we, you see, we were really frightfully poor ourselves—we were determined that, if we were to make a change in our people, then we should live no better than the poorest of them . . . "

"And so," continued Busuku, "I started to take in the kids; but we didn't have a nickel, and that's when I got the idea of the tax . . . "

"I mean it wasn't really a *tax* as such," corrected the Queen Mother.

"Blazes, Mother! Just let me tell it my way!" said Busuku defensively. "It *was* a tax, just the way I was brought up to design new taxes for the people. I mean, you get a good idea, and then you have to figure out how to *pay* for it, so you design a new *tax* for people to pay. I mean, Mother, that's the way government *works;* I mean, and I've said it before — that's what governments *do!*" Busuku huffed just a bit, out of breath, and then collected himself and went on.

"So I . . . you see . . . I design a tax, like any other Crown Prince. And it's called, you see, the Homeless Youth Self-Collection Tax. And the homeless boys, you see, they are sort of . . . you see . . . like tax collectors, that I trained to . . . well, you see . . . *collect the tax.*"

"They stole things," said the Queen Mother simply.

"Yes, well," and then the Prince glanced up at me, "although now of course I realize that this approach was creating the exactly opposite effect of what we intended. But oh well, anyway, one thing led to another and I began to spend a considerable amount of time as a . . . well, er, *guest* of this facility." His face got a little red; he wiped his chubby cheeks with a handkerchief and then went on quickly.

"But you see—parts of the master plan, they *were* in motion. I had sent several letters with caravans headed to Tibet, trying to re-establish contact with your uncle, the Maitri Pandita, himself—hoping he was still alive, hoping he could help us learn more about how yoga worked, you see, so we could pass it on up through the people.

"And then about a year ago—during another one of my extended stays here in the jail—the boys sneak in a letter: a reply from the Pandita himself. And it's the oddest letter . . ." He shook his head.

"Oh what did he say?" I gasped. "Is he well? Did he say anything of my family?"

Busuku . . . the Crown Prince . . . shook his head. "The letter said only that he fully understood the good things we hoped to do for our people, but that the Pandita was in no position himself to make the journey to the Realm. And then . . . strangest thing . . . he said that our needs had been . . . *foreseen* . . . he called it; and that a messenger had already been dispatched to us. And that she was a young Tibetan girl, of your description, travelling with a small dog, and that—now here's the oddest part—she doesn't *know* she's a messenger, and so we have to try to find this one girl among all the people passing through this town, and try to *delay* her until we can get some message out of her that she doesn't even know she's carrying. And somehow this message is going to be the key to bringing the people of our Realm all the health and happiness they could ever want.

"And so here I am locked up in this little mudbrick hole, and somehow I've got to make sure all the roads are covered night and day to intercept a messenger who doesn't know she's a messenger, and Mother is not someone who in her position and at her age could be outside standing on the roadside all day.

"So I send the boys to watch the smaller roads to the north and west, and I get the main road into town blocked off by the Sergeant, with his eye out for some 'precious contraband.'"

"But how did you know I was carrying the book?" I asked.

"I had no idea!" he exclaimed. "I just assumed, well—that you'd have *something* unusual with you; at least enough to get you to the jail for questioning. And you must know, Miss Friday . . . I had no idea that, well, some things would turn out so . . . so difficult here, or so long. And until yesterday I had no idea that you were the niece of the Pandita himself. And so I really am very sorry, and I beg your forgiveness for all the trouble we have caused you."

I waved my hand. "It was nothing, Bu . . . I mean, Your Highness. I think you realize that I . . . that I have stayed, because it was important to stay." And then I looked around at the three of them. "But as for a message . . . I have no idea what Uncle was thinking of; I have no message to give you."

Busuku smiled. "For many months I waited too for the message, and saw none; but then I realized what it was . . ." And at that moment the boys came running out the front door, laughing with excitement, glowing from their class with the Sergeant's son. We watched them through the screen, illuminated by the sunlight, and then they were gone around the back, to tend the corporal's orphans—and the new vegetable garden.

"And so the Crown Prince," continued the Superintendent then, "he wrote to me—just as the anonymous friend, you see—and told me that it would be in my interest, and in the interest of His Highness the King, if I could visit this station soon, and learn about what had changed the lives of people here so much. And so I have, and have reported too to His Highness, and received certain . . . instructions . . . back from him as well."

"Perhaps it is time . . . to begin passing those instructions on," said Busuku quietly, and he nodded towards the door of the station.

"With pleasure," smiled the Superintendent, and he rose and knelt again before the two. "Queen Mother," he said, and then "Crown Prince Dabi."

"*Busuku*, please," said Busuku. "Now, and forever after."

"Your Highness, Mr. . . Busuku," smiled the Superintendent again, and then he was gone.

I too began to get up, but the Queen Mother pressed my hand firmly in both her own. "One moment, please, Miss Friday," she said warmly, and then turned to address me. "There is . . . something more we wanted to speak to you about, in private."

I nodded, although to tell the true I had already heard more than enough to make my head spin. "Yes, of course, Queen Mother."

She laughed and touched my cheek with her hand. "And that's enough of that too! I am Amirta now, just the old lady Amirta, and like my son I choose to stay this way. Agreed?"

"Agreed," I smiled, "Amirta."

"That's better," she said, and then her voice took on a serious tone. "There is first of all something we want you to know, about my . . . friend, Mata Ji."

"The corporal's mother," I said.

"Ah yes," said Amirta, "and also my sister."

I smiled and hugged her. "But why didn't you tell me? What's the big secret?" I asked.

"It concerns her son," said the Queen Mother.

"You see, as first cousin to the new King, the corporal—when he turns thirty years of age, only a few years from now—becomes, by the laws of the Realm, the Prime Minister of this entire land, second only to the King himself."

Busuku studied my face while I worked this out, and giggled in delight when the shock hit me. "And you see, Miss Friday," he said then, "the corporal has no idea who he really is—and he must not know.

"Because, you see, this has been another key part of the master plan that Mother and I have been working on. We had a vision that the Prime Minister should be brought up among the common people—close to all their real problems, really understanding their needs, both as citizens and as . . . normal suffering creatures on this planet, born only to die. Things he would never learn at the royal court in the capital, until it was too late—until old age reached in through the luxury and comfort and began to strangle him.

"And we wanted him to be close to the Captain, you see," said Amirta, "so the seeds of the ideas that the Captain had heard from his own uncle as a young man would be planted early, just from personal contact."

"But we also had to be able to keep a close watch on him," said Busuku now. "Because, you see, the other factions—they are still strong, and terribly vigilant. If they had any idea of who we really are—and especially of who the corporal is, and will be—then our lives would be at immediate risk, out here in the countryside, so vulnerable. Even the Superintendent still has to travel with the guards, and he's added more people since he figured us out."

"And to be honest," said Amirta . . .

"Thank you, Mother," said Busuku . . .

"The Crown Prince *got* himself thrown in jail, so he

could keep an eye on the corporal, and make sure nothing happened to him," finished Amirta.

"But what you just said . . . about the tax for the boys and all . . . " I said.

"Was just for the Superintendent's benefit," said Busuku. "I mean, there *is* . . . I mean, *was* . . . a *tax*, you see, but it's not like I'd ever get *caught* collecting it; especially by a mere *sergeant*, if I didn't *try* to," he said proudly, with a glance at his mother.

"You see," she concluded, "no one must know that Mata Ji is my sister, or that the corporal is our next Prime Minister. Because part of our plan is that he must become *worthy* of the position: he must be challenged by the real world, and learn to cope with it himself, and develop here among the common people the real qualities that one needs to help lead them.

"We want to see if he can rise by himself, and in a sense it will be a test . . . a test of the message you have unknowingly brought us. I mean . . . will our dreams really come true, if we teach our young people that all things come from taking care of others?"

φ

The Captain and I both knew that events were boiling around us, and that our time could really be short now. But at our next class we both tried hard to thrust that out of our minds, and to concentrate. I felt a sadness but no regret; he had come to me like an empty vessel, and he was nearly full now. Only a few things remained to be said.

"We spoke about the milestones that come within your mind, as your garden reaches its fullness," I began. He nodded, and looked as though he wanted to say something—

383

perhaps many things, as did I. But right now this was most important, and we both knew it.

"There are milestones too even in your physical body," I went on, "and I thought that you should know about them . . . " I left the last part unsaid.

"Please," he said simply.

"Things will begin to change," I said, "as the new seeds from taking care of others begin to assert themselves; this happens even faster if you've been working to wipe out the old bad seeds . . . "

"I've been meaning to ask about that," he said then. "I mean, I guess it must be like waiting in line at the town well—everything moves faster if some people who got there earlier decide to leave, before they reach the front of the line."

"Exactly," I said, "which is why it's so important to work on the old bad seeds too. And then, you see, things with your body will begin to change. With most people, their own body is something they are blessed to see because of the very good seeds in their minds, from before. But like all seeds, good or bad, they wear out as they give their fruit."

"And that's why we see ourselves get older," he said simply.

"Just so," I said. "And because most people have no idea *why* they are getting older—no idea of what makes a pen a pen, no idea that it runs out of ink too only because *their* seeds have worn out—then they must simply go through the process helplessly, until the day they die.

"And in between there they may be fortunate enough to run into someone who can show them the yoga poses; and if they try them with some sincere regularity, then the choke-points around the middle channel are loosened, ever so slightly. And then for a while the aging slows down: they feel more energy, the joints open up.

"But if they don't understand where to go from there—if they don't really understand the power that the different forms of self-control have; if they don't understand that they can keep the seeds of their life from wearing out—then slowly, and very surely, they will continue to age, and there comes a time when yoga poses alone can no longer help.

"Someone who learns the Master's *Short Book* though—someone who learns the ideas we have spoken about, someone who begins to work on the seeds in their own mind, those who learn to garden—their life goes along a completely different path.

"They begin to do the poses, and the breathing exercises, and the silent sitting—giving and taking. And then very gradually and steadily they begin to feel a change in their very body. Sometimes they may not even be very much aware of it, because the change occurs from moment to moment, day and night; and since you are *in* your own body 24 hours a day, you don't notice the change the way, say, that a friend would who saw you only every few months.

"And so first the body gets lighter, the way it does at first with anyone who does the yoga poses. Then you begin to feel stronger, and you have much more energy. And then—as your purposeful changing of the seeds begins to affect the channels themselves—more fundamental changes occur. You begin to smell and taste things as you did when you were young, when the good seeds that gave you your body were still fresh. When you listen to a song you hear all the subtlety and hidden sweetness—an ability you had lost, as the years passed by, without even noticing it.

"And gradually the process builds upon itself; your bones themselves begin to grow younger, the back and neck become straight and supple again, you actually feel the flow of the good winds in your body, singing now, and you feel like dancing—like doing things you never dreamed of even when you were young.

"Here the balance of good and bad winds is shifting; you start to feel a certain steadiness of body and mind, as the turbulence within the side channels especially begins to slow. And in reflection of this you may even find your breath stopping for periods of time, quite unexpectedly. Quite certainly you will, as you progress, see the one most significant sign that the winds are shifting: a deep feeling simply of happiness; of contentment; of *peace* that continues throughout the day, every day. Things then are coming to the middle channel.

"And at the end, on the same day that your mind opens to all things, as we talked about before, well then your body too undergoes one final change. The very pattern of the channels themselves, around which your body originally grew, even in the womb, changes. The side channels collapse completely, for lack of any winds within them at all, for lack of any negative thoughts to ride there with them. All the energy of your very life and mind bursts into the middle channel, fully and forever. And then the body itself realigns itself to this new, most pure pattern. As the Master himself says,

> *You gain*
> *The body of perfection:*
> *A form of light itself;*
> *A frame of diamond strength.*
> III.47

And so your body becomes indestructible, like diamond itself, but living—perfect living crystal, shining in perfect light. No more flesh, no more bones or blood, through and through only perfect light. You can imagine it even now; the first seeds for it are within you even now, and you will look like what to you would be the most pure and innocent and lovely being you can imagine, although infinitely more so."

The Captain was staring up at me, entranced, and seeing as any of us would a tiny glimpse of what he would be. And then he looked up at me with the question I knew would come.

"Captain," I said, Katrin flowing through me. "See here; we spoke about it before. Throughout history there have been reports of miracles. I mean, maybe it's a woman in a boat with a few close friends on the great Ganges River. And she steps to the side of the boat, and out onto the water itself, and walks away upon it, some distance from the boat, and turns, and stands there, with her arms open wide.

"And you see, it is all because of the seeds in her own mind. In that sense it is no miracle at all; it is the simple result of patient, dedicated gardening of the seeds within her own mind. She has perfected the art of self-control: she is perfect in never harming a single other living creature.

"And the water is helping, you see: it is being a perfect helper, because—like the pen—it is *not* being *itself*. *Water is not wet by itself*: it is only the seeds in *our* minds that make us see it so. And her seeds, you see, they are *different*: they are *perfect*. And when she looks down at the water, when *she* steps upon it, it is as solid as marble itself.

"But what of her friends in the boat? One or two may have seeds to *make* the same miracle, if only for a few steps. The others though, all of them, *have seeds in their mind that are still so pure* that they are able to *witness* a miracle taking place. And you must understand that—if it requires perfect seeds to *make* a miracle—then it needs only slightly *less* perfect seeds to *witness* one being made." I paused to see if he would tie it together.

The Captain gazed out the window, in a sort of rapture. "What you're saying," he said softly, "is what I was wondering. I mean, someone like the corporal say—he could finish all his gardening a week from now. Goodness, for all we know, he could have finished it years ago. And to *himself*, when *he* looks in a mirror, he sees then a perfect body of diamond light. And to *us*, for those of us who are just beginning to garden perhaps, he looks like a normal person, of mortal flesh and blood. And we will not see him as anything more than that . . . "

" . . . until we come closer to changing into that ourselves," I finished.

"And so the fact that we have not seen angels—that we have not seen those who came before and used the Master's book, or any other such book, to change themselves . . . "

"Doesn't prove a thing," I concluded, "about whether they really exist or not. Ask any cow . . . "

"About the existence of . . . ," he added.

"Pens!" we both cried out, and we leaned over the desk and hugged each other, as if we would never have another chance.

47

Grace

First Week of February

A few nights later, when everyone had gone to bed on time for once, Crown Prince Busuku's voice came in the dark to me, softly.

"Miss Friday," he said quietly. "Are you still awake?"

"I am," I replied. Long-Life and I always stayed up a little later, to snuggle at night and watch the stars out the window.

"Ah good," he said, and then he was silent for a moment. "Because," he continued then, with a sadness in his voice, "there is one more thing that I haven't told you about yet."

"Yes?" I said, sitting up with worry beginning to grow inside me.

"It's about . . . it's about the letter I received from your uncle," he said, "over a year ago."

"Yes?" I said again, my heart pounding. Perhaps something had happened to Mother?

"At the end of the letter, you see, there was something else . . . he said it was 'a message to the messenger, when her message has been delivered.' And I suppose . . . I suppose now it's really all been delivered, you see . . . "

"Yes," I said, "I think nearly all of it, now."

"Ah yes," he said sadly, and was quiet again. "Well . . . it said," and his voice again began to break, "it said that 'the best teachers find themselves becoming the pupil again,' and then there was . . . there was something about a stream, or a river, you see . . .

"That's all," he said abruptly.

I looked out at the stars, and thought of all the people out there among them, and I said simply, "I understand, my Prince."

φ

It was hard going keeping up with the Superintendent's huge strides, and the Captain wasn't faring much better.

"Surprise!" he called back to us heartily. "I always like it to be a surprise! And I like the whole family to be there too!" He covered another forty feet of a pasture out west, behind the jail, and then stopped and threw his palms to his chest. "Ah, the morning air in the country! You can't imagine how good it smells, after the Capital!" We caught up, puffing, and walked three abreast.

"Now I ask you one more time, Kishan," said the Superintendent to the Captain. "You're sure . . . that the Sergeant had nothing to do with those false reports and all."

"Nothing at all," replied the Captain gravely. "It was all my own doing, sir."

"And no other problems that he's ever had that . . . that might prevent him from fulfilling the duties successfully?"

I glanced at the Captain. He seemed under some kind of intense strain. I had no idea what was going on, but both the Captain and I knew very well that with a few words now he could ruin the Sergeant forever. The Captain caught my eye for a split-second and then said, "Nothing at all, sir, nothing at all. An exemplary officer, in both his official and his family life."

"Excellent," replied the Superintendent. "Then that's that," and we marched on, to the Sergeant's house.

And the Captain and I stood back near the neat little gate, while the Superintendent strode across the well-kept grass and knocked at the door. And we saw the Sergeant open it, and he was all bright and chipper and freshly washed and dressed neat as a pin, and the morning sun beamed in upon his smiling face, and on the lovely faces of his wife and his boy standing at his side, all looking as if they had just finished their poses and their sitting—which I suppose they had.

And the Superintendent booms out "Greetings to you all on this glorious day," and with warm hands he pushes a letter into the Sergeant's hands. And the Sergeant opens it, and nearly falls down with joy and surprise, for it is an official correspondence from the Ministry of Justice, proclaiming him the new captain of the station.

And I feel the Captain next to me—I feel the heart in his chest—and it is about to break, but he smiles bravely and waves his congratulations to the Sergeant and his family; and the Sergeant's face clouds over for a moment, asking the Captain if things are all right; and the Captain dismisses it cheerfully with a little brush of his hand in the air, and the smile returns to the Sergeant's face. And then we are walking back to the station, in a silence that feels like a funeral, and we stop in a little cluster of trees way out behind the jail.

The Superintendent froze then, always wary, and kept us back in the cover of the shadows, under the trees. "Look there," he said softly. "Coming across the field there."

A huge shaft of morning light slanted across the brilliant green of the field, and we could see a lone man leading a horse.

"Odd," said the Superintendent, straining his eyes against the light.

"What's that?" whispered the Captain.

"Lame," said the Superintendent. "Badly lame." And we could see that the horse was limping with every step. "Who would keep a horse like that?" mused the Superintendent. "Uses up a bag of feed every day, and can't do a lick of work."

The Captain looked at me suddenly, and we shielded our eyes with our hands and saw that, yes, it was the corporal—sneaking another abandoned animal into the pasture behind the jail.

"Uh, it's the corporal, sir," said the Captain awkwardly.

"The corporal? Our corporal?"

"Yes sir."

"But . . . why the horse? Why keep a useless horse?"

"He, sir . . . ," the Captain paused, and I gave him a Grandmother look. No use planting a bad seed by lying now, of all times.

"He takes in animals that have been abandoned, sir. Takes care of them, you see, out behind the jail."

The Superintendent turned and appraised the Captain briefly, and then turned back to mark the slow progress of the pair across the field.

They reached the embankment that sloped to the stream far behind the back of the jail. It was steep and muddy, and the crippled mare shied back, looking down with big frightened eyes, pulling on the rope.

"Come now, come," said the corporal softly. "No need to worry, pretty one. Almost home now." And he started down the slope slowly, working against the rope.

The horse threw her head back with a violent jerk that tore the rope from the corporal's hand, and he flew backwards down the slope, landing in a length of mud at the side of the stream. He lay there still as death, and we held our breath waiting.

And then the corporal gets up with a little sigh, and he stands up to his ankles in the mud, and he twists around to see the backside of his fresh white cotton trousers, and the whole back of his crisp new white shirt, covered with a slick black mud.

And he looks up at her and spreads his arms wide to the sky and says, "So much for impressing the Superintendent!" And he steps up the embankment to her and laughs like a song and takes her huge grey head in his arms and hugs it against his chest, and fills the sky with his laughter. And the song settles her heart, and he throws his arm around her neck, and they walk slowly down the slope, side by side.

The Superintendent stood stock-still with his mouth open, watching the scene. "Such humility," he whispered, "such compassion." And then he turned around to the Captain and me.

"After all these years running the Ministry," he said, "I've learned only one thing about people. You can teach almost anyone to do any job—goodness, almost any fool there could even do my own job; I mean, the technical stuff. But to find a man with true humility, a man with real compassion—things that are so very difficult to *cultivate* in another person who doesn't already have them—now *that* is a treasure." He looked back at the corporal and the mare, making their way across the stream now. "And I'm not getting any younger either," he said to himself.

And then suddenly he leaped ahead out of the bushes. "Stay here for a while if you don't mind," he called over his shoulder. "Just until I've had a word or two with the corporal."

"Yes . . . sir," said the Captain in a despondent tone.

The Superintendent whirled around, still walking—backwards—and exclaimed, "And oh, Captain! Please try not to be so glum!" The Captain looked after him glumly, and glanced to his side, at me.

"Lost everything," he called back. "Even my Teacher."

The Superintendent stopped, and they continued their conversation yelling over the breadth of half a pasture.

"Nonsense!" he yelled. "*She's* losing *you!*"

The Captain looked confused. "But the other day—in the station. You said there would be a lot of changes: you said the yoga teacher would have to go to the Capital; help you and the King himself learn yoga by the book, by the *Short Book*; and then go out to all the other stations, and help make them like ours."

"It's *you* that's going to the capital!" bellowed the Superintendent, casting a worried glance at the slowly drying black of the corporal's back, disappearing now over the other side of the stream.

The Captain's eyes glazed over in shock. "Am I to be imprisoned then?" he cried.

The Superintendent took three huge strides back towards us, his big hands clenched in frustration at his sides. "Blazes, Captain. You're so blasted *thick* for a Captain, or even an ex-Captain! Living at the King's side may be a pain, but it's hardly a prison! You're coming to the capital *to be the teacher!* Teacher to all of us!"

The Captain gulped, and then looked up at the sky in wonder, and then to me with a worried expression. "Not to worry about her!" called the Superintendent with a mighty laugh, and he started walking backwards to the station again. "Miss Friday continues on to Varanasi, to the banks of the holy Ganges! Meets old and very, very wise friends of her uncle and aunt—I know just where they are! All her dreams come true!"

And with this the Superintendent turned and started jogging after the corporal. "And of course the two of you meet again later on, and do some terribly wonderful and compassionate deeds together to help . . . " and a wind flew up and threw his last words around our heads like a chain of flowers " . . . all the rest of us!" And he was gone.

φ

It was a little odd sitting across from the Captain's desk at our next class. He had insisted that the Sergeant move in right away, and everyone had taken the opportunity to carry all the old reports out back and burn them in a big beautiful fire in the evening. The room was bright now, with freshly whitewashed walls, and a newly finished painting hung in a frame up behind the Captain's head. A man from town had come and done it in a day: a group portrait of all the boys, along with Busuku and Amirta and Mata Ji; and me holding Long-Life up against my chest; and right in the middle the Superintendent, with his huge arms around the shoulder of the Captain on one side, and the Sergeant and the corporal on the other. Our whole family.

"The Captain said we had to use his room, right up to the last day," said the Captain.

"He's been so good," I nodded, and we fell silent for a moment, like the old days.

"We spoke about milestones within your own mind," I began softly, "and then we spoke about them with your body—about the change." He nodded as he always did, and I looked again at the handsome black curls of his hair, the way I had the first day—things you never notice if you think you'll always be with someone.

"But there are other changes," I went on, my throat feeling all tight now. "And it's good if you hear about them too, and then you'll know—when you see them—that you are on the right track; that your gardening is coming along well.

"You see, it's not just the inside of you that changes. Things around you begin to change too—people, events, the very place that you live in. The Master reveals this change in lines like the following:

> *If you make it a way of life*
> *Never to hurt others,*
> *Then in your presence*
> *All conflict comes to an end.*
>
> II.35

And it's a *principle* he's talking about; and there's a truth behind the principle," I said.

"The truth goes back to what we said a long time ago—about how things grow like layers of ice forming around the contours of a twig.

"We have a certain pattern of thoughts; we *think* in certain patterns: we *misunderstand* ourselves and the world around us, in certain typical ways, even from the first moment in the womb.

"And then that subtle network of channels deep within us forms, assuming the same faulty pattern of our thoughts—thoughts which then run in the channels, riding on the winds there, for the rest of our lives. And just as the thoughts are twisted, in a way—'turning things around the wrong way,' as the Master would say—then the side channels twist around the middle channel, creating the choke-points.

"And then our bodies form around the pattern of these channels, with crucial sections of our bones and nerves and blood vessels themselves situated at their important junctures: those centers of energy we call the *chakras*, restricted severely by the side channels. And that much we've talked about at length," I said. The Captain nodded once more, following closely. I wondered for a moment if there wasn't any way to get *every* class to feel like the last class—death could always make it so, and so any class *could* be the last—and it did wonders for the student's attention span.

"But there's more, you see; the layers don't end there. Because the entire world around us *forms then around the faulty pattern of the channels*; I'm talking about *all the things you will ever see*, in your whole life; and all the places you ever 'go' to; and all the people you ever meet; and every event that happens around you—whether it's close enough to touch with your hand, or away around the other side of the globe, or among or beyond the stars themselves. EVERYTHING IS A REFLECTION OF THE CONDITION OF YOUR OWN HEART; or at least of the condition of your garden: of the seeds you have planted there, by being kind or not to others.

"And so looking at the world is like looking in a funny kind of mirror—a mirror that takes weeks or months or even longer to reflect your face back to you after you step in front of it."

The Captain gazed at me fervently. "Incredible," he said simply. "And so obviously true, if all that we have said about seeds making us see things is true: if the simple fact of the pen and the cow is true, as we know it must be. I mean, it's one thing to comprehend suddenly that if I meet a bad person it is really only all my own fault: seeds in my own mind, planted by *me*, going off and making me see them that way—the same way that seeds make me, but not the cow, see the green stick as a pen.

"But to imagine that *every single thing* in my world is the same; to imagine that every single instance of conflict in my world—from an unkind word that someone says to me on the road in the morning, all the way up to massive international wars that are fought within my lifetime, anywhere in the world—to imagine that *their very existence* depends on the state of *my own channels*, of *my own thoughts*, flowing within me . . . " He staggered into a kind of silence, and then looked up at me, as I knew he would.

"Yes, others experience them too—I mean, the wars. Three people can sit in a room, and another person walks in; two of them can experience these latest shapes and colors as a very irritating person. But the third . . . "

The Captain shook his head like an upset bull. "But a *war*; my goodness. A *war!* Are you telling me that a million people can be embroiled in a conflict which threatens their very world, while there are other people, *living in the same place*, who experience it as something completely different? Even . . . ," he choked on the thought.

" . . . even as, say, heaven?" I asked, and I reached down on the desk and pulled the pen up between us one last time.

"And this is exactly what the Master is saying in this exquisite line," I whispered intensely. "It is why he says 'in *your* presence,' don't you see? In *your* world, as *your* seeds make it: existing within and alongside of *other people's* worlds, as *their* seeds make *them*. The green stick is a pen; the same stick is something to eat; all at the same time, but to two different people.

"Oh Captain, don't you see? You once asked me why the side channels were named 'Sun' and 'Moon'—you were thinking that perhaps the sun and the moon have some special influence upon them—but now you see . . . " I paused.

"That they . . . that they *create* the sun and the moon? Layers of ice on ice, even that . . . even that far?" he cried. We were silent for a long time, and then he chuckled and shook his head. "So when those two channels die out—what will we use for light?"

"The light of heaven comes from the bodies of those who live there," I said simply, and gave him some time to imagine it.

"But it doesn't come all at once, you see," I said then, "and that's why I wanted to tell you more . . . more about what to expect, along the way.

"You see now *how* it works—which is how yoga itself works, really—and so you see the truth behind the principle: the principle that, if you sincerely try to avoid harming others, then all conflict disappears from the entire world you experience.

"But the same principle applies to every other form of goodness that you could ever do: to all the other forms of self-control; to giving and taking and to all the other kinds of infinite good thoughts that we talked about. All together they have an effect on your world: they *make* your *new* world.

"Watch for it now, Captain; watch for it now. She comes in four different stages, you can say, and if you are watching carefully you will see them coming — otherwise they will just happen to you, and you may not even notice it; since really it is *you* that is changing, and the rest is only your reflection.

"The first step is called Noticeable. I mean, your life is rolling along like before, but you're consciously *trying* to put all that we've talked about into actual practice, within your own everyday life. And then small things start to happen, you see—small, but noticeable. Your walk to work is a little more pleasant on one day, and then on the next—and the next: too many to be a complete accident. There are more nice people on the road. More people smile at you and bid you good morning.

"And then secondly, a little further on, you see, comes the Surprising. You go to work one day and your employer, who is frankly known to be a little tight-fisted, sits you down; tells you what a fine job you're doing; and gives you a considerable raise in salary, just like that. The effects of the work you've done on your own seeds—your gardening—graduate from noticeable to surprising.

"And then thirdly there is the Amazing: I mean, something that's not totally impossible, but only slightly less so. Say you decide to look for a bigger place to make a school, for more homeless children. And then a few days later you are standing in a line at a shop, and a lady mentions that her aunt is hoping to donate an entire estate—acres and acres of valuable land, and a beautiful house—to a worthy charity. And, amazingly, it becomes that new school.

"And then finally you see there comes the clearly Impossible. You and a friend go tomorrow to a strange city—to a place where you know no one. You walk down a street at random, and go into a small café. A pleasant older woman serves the two of you a fine meal—a rather expensive meal. And when you ask the woman for the bill she steps back abruptly, and says with surprise, "Really now! Do you think we would accept money from a person who is about to introduce the Master's *Short Book* to so many people?" And with that she simply walks away. Something has happened which is . . . impossible, in the normal world.

"And Captain, of all the lessons I have taught to you, this is perhaps the most important. And this I tell you: When these things come to you, and they will, then it is very important how you respond to them. It is a crucial moment for the seeds in your mind that will trigger the final changes within you—the ones that turn you to light, the ones that open your mind to all things, the ones that enable you to see and to go to countless people in countless worlds, all at the same time, and bring them on to ultimate happiness. And all you need to do in that moment, in the moment that the old woman, or whoever she may be—and it could be a stranger, or a friend, or a husband, or a wife, or mother, father, or child—in the moment that they come to you, bringing the impossible to you, you must only have faith, and believe in them totally. Do not seek an explanation, lest it come and kill the magic. Even if all you get is a glimpse—even if only for a single minute a single person says or does something to you which could even suggest that *they are already the being of light which you seek to be*—then accept it as so, wholly. Have faith, do not doubt, and that faith will quickly bring you amongst them. For there are truly countless holy ones who have travelled the path you have learned here, long before us. They swarm around our sadness and the mortality of us like bees clustered upon a sweet flower, striving to teach us, striving to be seen, striving to free us to be with them.

"And so as you do your gardening, watch for them. And never, ever, ever, disappoint them when they grant you a glimpse of their face. Accept in that moment their grace—all the grace they seek to give you—with complete and final grace."

48

Your Hand

Second Week of February,
Water Horse Year (1102 A.D.)

Busuku and the boys' surprise breakfast party was a wild affair; this time it was the Superintendent who took off his shirt and danced, as he was already beginning to feel the effects of his first few yoga sessions. (He had been sneaking into the boys' class in the mornings.)

But now the sadness of parting could no longer be pushed away; the soldiers were outside with the Superintendent's wagon, loading it with the last of the Captain's things, for the trip back to the capital. The corporal—or rather, the new Deputy Assistant Superintendent of the Ministry of Justice—was deep in conversation with the Superintendent, up in the side room. He and one of the Superintendent's men were to be my escorts to Varanasi, and he was getting last-minute instructions on the route, along with letters of introduction to those who had helped my aunt and uncle in their own quest. We were to travel on foot, for I had refused a coach or even horses: one must approach one's Teacher humbly.

I picked up my old shoulder bag, with all I owned in it; gathered Long-Life into my arms; and looked around at my cell one last time. In a sense, the world had truly come to it, seeking its freedom. I stepped out.

"Prisoner attempting to escape!" roared Official School (Jail) Principal—that was how they decided to write it in the end—Master Busuku. And he ran and caught me in his arms and gave me one last big hug; and then there was a long line of hugs from all the rest, from the Sergeant (Captain) down to the last little boy, and the Superintendent, and there at the end in the sunlight of the doorway was the Captain. And he was crying openly and he called out, "Only a moment please" to the others, and took my hand and pulled me into his old office, and shut the door behind us.

"Your book," he said, and handed me an exquisitely wrapped little package.

"But I have it here," I replied, tapping my shoulder bag. "You gave it back to me last week."

"Ah, not the old book, and the notes of the classes that my Teacher had with her own dear Teacher. This is a record of our own classes—of every class you ever taught me." And I looked up at his tears and burst into my own.

"We have made copies, for the others to come . . . ," he added lamely, at a loss for words.

"Then they shall be incomplete," I smiled as best I could, and pulled him down to the desk one last time.

"One more change you have to know about," I said quickly. "We've talked about how your body will change— about how it becomes like living light. But that's just the body that you *live* in. On the day that all the final changes take place, you gain an infinite number of other physical forms. The Master describes them like this:

The bodies that you send out
Come only from your thoughts,
And from the true nature
Of yourself.

IV.4

And we have talked about it ever since the first days that you began to do yoga to help your back—we said it could never work if you did it only for yourself. And so each day before we practiced the poses we did the silent sitting, and we imagined our breath—the same breath we were about to carry to the poses—going out, and taking away someone's pain. And then with that same breath we gave them everything they could ever wish for, up to freedom from death itself. And you have seen, with the Sergeant and the corporal, how thought itself becomes reality.

"And then later we made the thought bigger; we imagined helping countless people, in countless worlds, all at the same time: we made the thought *infinite*. And we talked about having this thought even as you practice the yoga poses—for it is the very *goal* of the poses.

"And on that final day, a split-second after your mind opens to see all things in all time—all within a single tiny point—you suddenly send forth your new forms: your new bodies, to every place where people wait for you; for now you see them all before you.

"And it's not a conscious thought, you see—you make no decision to go forth to all worlds. It simply *happens*, by the power of your new state of mind, and by the power of all the thoughts, all the seeds you planted in the past — ever since the first day you sat down to think of helping the Sergeant.

405

"And this is why you must *always* begin your poses with the silent sitting, giving and taking: with thoughts of helping someone you know—and eventually of helping everyone there is. Because on that day it is these seeds that will send you forth—you in countless shapes and forms—to stand at the side of every living creature in whatever likeness they personally can relate to at that moment; to help them along a little further, every single day they have left before they themselves can send forth these forms, to others.

"And send them forth they will, for it is the greatest miracle of all, that each of us must become the one savior of every world there is."

He looked up at me.

"And why is it this way? I leave you with that last question—you will understand it from those last words of the Master's, and from this."

I picked up the pen from his desk, and held it up between us.

"Dear pen," he said, and he reached out and touched it, and his hand was pure light.

"Your hand!" I cried; and "Your hand!" he cried.

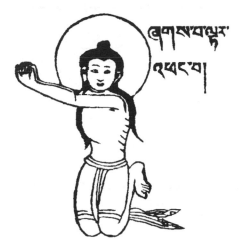

As you can tell, *How Yoga Works* is not just a story. The wisdom here is taken straight from the ancient books of Tibet and India, and it works as well today as it did a thousand years ago. You can actually use it to make your body young and strong, and your heart open and happy. If you'd like to learn more about studying this ancient knowledge and learning to practice it yourself, please visit the Yoga Studies Institute at www.yogastudiesinstitute.org. We'd be happy to help you.